Out of my
Valley

Alice Fletcher

Out of my Valley

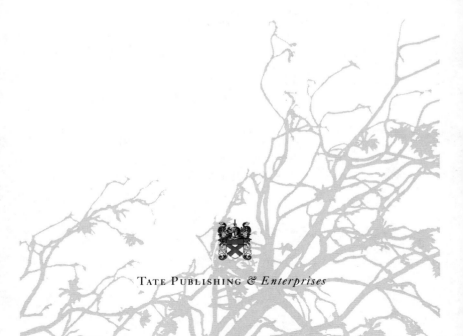

a cancer survivor's journey
to meaning and hope

Tate Publishing & *Enterprises*

Published by Tate Publishing & Enterprises, LLC
127 E. Trade Center Terrace | Mustang, Oklahoma 73064 USA
1.888.361.9473 | www.tatepublishing.com

Tate Publishing is committed to excellence in the publishing industry. The company reflects the philosophy established by the founders, based on Psalm 68:11,
"The Lord gave the word and great was the company of those who published it."

Book design copyright © 2009 by Tate Publishing, LLC. All rights reserved.
Cover design by Amber Gulilat
Interior design by Blake Brasor

Published in the United States of America

ISBN: 978-1-60799-427-5
1. Biography & Autobiography / Personal Memoirs
2. Religion / Christian Life / Inspirational
09.06.03

Some of the proceeds from the selling of this book will be donated to the American Cancer Society for research on all types of cancer.

Dedication

This book is dedicated to Ed, my husband, for his love, provision, leadership, and protection during our forty-five years of marriage to date.

The following poems and narrative are dedicated to the following:

"My Invisible Friend" is dedicated to Marianne King, my friend and sister in the Lord. The Lord knew I needed a special friend here on earth to walk through the valley with me as we walked together with our Invisible Friend.

"Listen to God" is dedicated to Terry Aldridge, my current Sunday school teacher, for his series of lessons on *Listen to God*, which inspired me to write the poem.

"Reach Out and Touch Him" is dedicated to our sons, Mike, Clay, Clint, and Luke, for their love, prayers, and concerns for "Momma" during my deep valley and always.

"Our Christian Journey" is dedicated to Clay and Kacey.

While going through their valley, I felt inspired to pen these words down.

"Where the Lilies Grow" is dedicated to Dr. Charles E. Wright, a devout man full of wisdom, who during a sermon many years ago said, "Lilies grow in the valley, not on the mountaintop." I will always remember this.

"Don't Let the Stones Cry Out" is dedicated to Don Marks, my brother, who is going through a valley now. It was written to emphasize to him that in all things we can give thanks and praise; it is attainable.

Acknowledgments

The greatest thanks is to my Savior, the Lord Jesus Christ, the great three in one. "For there are three that bear record in heaven, the Father, the Word, and the Holy Ghost: and these three are one" (1 John 5:7). All glory and praise to my Lord and Savior for his virgin birth, his sacrificial death on Calvary, his burial, and his resurrection to become my living Savior; leaving with us his infallible written Word for an example on how to live a victorious life, one that will be pleasing to him. The Bible is for our instruction, correction, and communication with him.

It is with extreme gratitude I thank the Lord with all my being for the guidance and teaching I have received from all the pastors I have had since the day of my salvation. Those being Rev. Darrell Hayes; Rev. Doyle Conley; Dr. Charles E. Wright; Dr. David A. McCoy; and my present pastors, Rev. Brandon Brooks and senior pastor Dr. Charles W.

Chapman. If it were not for their teaching and expounding on the Scriptures, I would not have been able to write this book. It is through their faithfulness in preaching that I have grown spiritually. "So then faith cometh by hearing, and hearing by the word of God" (Romans 10:17).

I thank my husband, Ed, for his faithfulness and leadership while traveling along our Christian journey together during these thirty-eight years. I truly believe if it had not been for his salvation a few months prior to me receiving Christ, I might not be a Christian today. I saw such a change in him; I knew there was something he had that I needed.

With great appreciation I express thanks to Don Marks, my brother, for the time he spent reading and making corrections to my manuscript. He had a big job on his hands!

Many thanks to Clint Fletcher, our son, for spending a day of his time searching the Internet and making telephone calls for me in my desperation for a new computer.

Words are not adequate enough to express my sincere thanks to Ginger Fletcher, our daughter-in-law, for her enormous blessing to me. My new computer was not compatible with the program on the old one, therefore she insisted on typing the entire book over for me. Ginger is a wife, mother, and works full time. Only God knows my heart, as thanks is not enough.

Thanks to Don Marks; Jan Marks; Jan's friend, Brenda Reynolds; and Jane Marks for their words of encouragement after reading my manuscript.

Table of Contents

 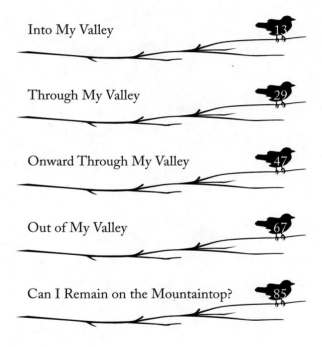

Into My
Valley

It was a beautiful mid-autumn day in the year of our Lord 2005. I had completed my morning school bus route and was on my way to a doctor's appointment. Having had a breast biopsy two weeks prior, this was a return appointment for the results. One would usually return in one week, but Dr. Mattison was on vacation the week following my biopsy.

I went alone, not having a thought of an unfavorable report. I had had two breast biopsies in the past, and both were benign. Although the one in 1987 was benign, I had a lumpectomy to remove the cyst because of the location and discomfort it caused. The second biopsy was just the previous year, in October 2004, in the same area of question. I had my yearly mammograms on schedule.

On that Monday, November 7, Dr. Mattison gave me

the dreaded words no one wants to hear. I had breast cancer. The pathology report stated that the cancer did not originate in my breast. This added news was overwhelming. Dr. Mattison ordered a PET scan for the next day and scheduled an appointment to return to his office the following week.

As I walked through the valley of the shadow, back to my car, the Lord gave me a scripture I needed at that very moment, not realizing at first the great impact it was going to have on my life. I thought how strange for this particular scripture that God so tenderly spoke in his still, small voice that only my heart heard, to come to me at that very moment; after all, let's face it, I had just received troubling news. "... for I have learned, in whatsoever state I am, therewith to be content" (Philippians 4:11). A few moments later, after the shock, it came to mind that this was God's way of reminding me I have choices, choices on how I could handle this situation. He was conveying to me to not go to pieces but to depend on him. I was already setting myself up for one gigantic pity party, but God intervened in such a marvelous way that my pity party had to go by the wayside. Sometimes we dwell on ourselves and want to wallow in a good pity party, which I know is not pleasing to the Lord. Sitting in my car trying to absorb this news, I felt God gently blow the cloud of fear away. Had I not been obedient to his still, small voice, I hate to conceive of what state of mind I would have found myself.

Unexplainable peace came over me while sitting there in a meditative, motionless state. "And the peace of God, which passeth all understanding, shall keep your hearts and minds through Christ Jesus" (Philippians 4:7). "Thou wilt keep him in perfect peace, whose mind is stayed on thee: because he trusteth in thee" (Isaiah 26:3). He gave me complete assurance that he would be with me through this deep valley.

I called Ed, my husband, from my cell phone. He was on a job and I hated to give him this news over the phone, but knowing him, he would want to know immediately. He was speechless for a few moments then said, "I am almost finished with the inspection, and I will be home as quickly as I can get there."

While driving home another scripture came to me. "The Lord is my shepherd; I shall not want. He maketh me to lie down in green pastures ..." (Psalm 23:1–2). I shall never forget the day this scripture became so clear to me. In the late 1970s I was sitting at our kitchen table studying to teach a ladies' Bible study group, and I was looking out the window across the pasture. I noticed all the cows were lying down chewing their cud. The Lord so tenderly showed me how content and peaceful the cows were. It was late spring and the pasture was lush and green. After they had grazed in the morning, had eaten enough, and were satisfied, they were lying down in green pastures. Had they chosen not to graze on what was available for them, I would have heard them bellowing as they sometimes do in the winter when Ed works overtime and is late for feeding time.

Oh, how peaceful and content the Christian life is when we allow the Lord to feed us daily from his Holy Word, our Bread of Heaven. I sometimes wonder how much of God's Word a Christian has been feasting on when I hear them bellowing. The Lord knows that we are going to go through difficulties even before we get there. He yearns for us to depend on him for strength to walk with him through them. Don't take me wrong; our initial feelings are ones of question, worry, and why me? If we dwell on the things God has taught us from the Bible, we will soon see our way out of that state of mind and enter into a state of peace, as we realize our Lord is allowing this and will walk each step of the way with us.

I thought of Dan Harden, a wonderful, dedicated Christian man, who in early 1970 was instrumental in leading Ed to the Lord and several months later led me to the Lord. I thought of him often, and my thoughts always turned to thanking the Lord for his witness. The day Dan showed me the way to salvation, he gave me a Bible verse to memorize. He called throughout the week to encourage me to read the Bible daily, asking if I had any questions on the scriptures I had read. He invited our family to attend church with his family the following Sunday and go home with them for dinner. We were already actively attending a local church, and I was teaching Sunday school, but neither Ed nor I had personally accepted Jesus Christ as our Savior.

After church services and a wonderful dinner with the Hardens, we sat and fellowshipped with the family. Before we left to attend evening services with them, Mr. Harden asked me to recite the verse he had given to me. "There hath no temptation taken you but such as is common to man: but God is faithful, who will not suffer you to be tempted above that ye are able; but will with the temptation also make a way to escape, that ye may be able to bear it" (1 Corinthians 10:13). He gave me another verse to memorize for the next week.

A few years later, Helen, Dan's wife, phoned to ask if she

could enroll our sons in Bible Memory Association. What a magnificent program for memorizing Bible verses. The program was designed for ages three to a hundred and three. After our children had been in the program two years, the Lord convicted me to memorize Bible verses with them. I should not have them do something I was not doing. The verses I have hidden in my heart have come to memory during difficult times and happy times over the years, just as the Holy Spirit was faithful in bringing them to me at this needed hour. The verses that came to memory on the day I received my cancer report gave me satisfaction to my soul.

Ed arrived home from his job just minutes before I had to leave to begin my afternoon school bus route. We talked about my cancer and how I had not even imagined receiving such news. We knew our sons needed to know but decided not to telephone them until we learned more from the PET scan. Off I went for the three-hour excursion.

Upon returning home, Ed said, "Clint said he would be there tomorrow for the PET scan." Sometime later he told me he had talked with Mike and Luke but had not been able to reach Clay yet.

I replied, "I thought we had determined not to tell the boys anything until we found out the extent of the cancer."

He felt they needed to know immediately. It eased his mind some to have the boys share in this. He didn't have to carry the burden alone! He had also called our preacher and several friends. He must have spent the entire three hours on the telephone.

The next day, Ed and I arrived at the office for my PET

scan. Our son Clint drove into the parking lot at the same time we did. I was to arrive early to fill out paperwork and drink a solution thirty minutes before being taken back to a preparation room. Shortly after we arrived, another son, Luke, and his wife, Alisia, came into the waiting room. We sat and talked for thirty minutes. After the time had elapsed, the nurse called my name to go with her. All five of us stood up, and the nurse acted as if she did not know what to say.

After a moment, she said, "Only two others can go with you."

Of course that meant Ed and one son. Clint and Luke looked at each other as if to say, *Put up your dukes and start with one potato, two potato, three potato, four, five potato, six potato, seven potato, or; etc.*; this was a formality they did as kids to determine who would go first in a game or who would be it in tag.

The nurse looked at each of us and said, "Okay, all right, all of you can come on back."

There the six of us were, crammed into a small preparation room. She explained the procedure and what to expect; then she injected a radiation tracker into a vein in my arm and asked everyone else to leave the room. I had to remain in a quiet, darkened room for one hour for the radiation tracker to circulate throughout my body before the scan could be done. I was sitting in a comfortable recliner during this time praying and being thankful that Clint, Luke, and Alisia had taken the time from their schedule to come support us.

After the hour was up, I was taken into the machine room for the scan. I had to lie down on a table, and my whole body was moved into the machine and back out very slowly. The scan was taking images from my head to my feet and took approximately forty-five minutes. I had to wait to get the results of the scan when I returned to Dr. Mattison's office the next week. I must confess, I found myself worrying, wondering where else in my body the cancer could be. Then this thought came to me: *Where is the peace I had yesterday?*

A past pastor, Dr. Charles Wright, frequently said, "Worry is like rocking in a rocking chair; it will give you something to do but will get you nowhere."

I realized then that I was in a win-win situation. Living would allow me to remain on earth; death would take me home to heaven. Sure, death would separate me from my loved ones, but it would be as though I changed my residence and they could move and join me there later, if they also had eternal life in Jesus Christ. Why worry? I realized that although the verses on peace and contentment came to me, I had not been obedient to the commandment. "Casting all your care upon him; for he careth for you" (1 Peter 5:7).

Laying this cancer at his feet at that moment through prayer, the peace that passeth all understanding returned to me again.

Wednesday of that week, just three days later, as I woke to start my day, the Lord laid on my heart a thought that just astonished me. Before my feet hit the floor, this thought came to me: *I have an Invisible Friend.* I had a mental picture of my Lord walking hand in hand with me. Before the week was over, the Lord gave me words to a poem that has stayed with me and helped me tremendously along this road through my valley. I know this was from the Lord, as I had never written anything previously.

About ten months later, my Sunday school teacher read the following verse during his lesson: "Now unto the King eternal, immortal, invisible, the only wise God, be honour and glory forever and ever. Amen" (1 Timothy 1:17).

I sat there amazed and said to myself, "Glory to God, my Invisible Friend."

There are other verses that portray God as invisible. "Who is the image of the invisible God, the firstborn of every creature" (Colossians 1:15), speaking of Jesus, part of the Trinity.

Out of my Valley

My Invisible Friend

When I was just a wee little child
And all my needs were met, I felt secure.
My thoughts were only for the present day,
Not for my eternal life, that's for sure.

Then in my teens, as I was spreading
My wings and feeling oh so carefree,
I had a loving family and many a friend,
But I mainly dwelt on me.

And one day one knocked on my
Heart's door wanting to be my friend.
He touched my heart, convicted me of my sin,
And in repentance I welcomed him in.

It was on that day when I accepted Jesus
As my Savior and he became my friend,
That I read in his word that the Holy Spirit
Came into my life and shall ever abide within.

As I grow older and face the trials
And tribulations of life that come my way,
My Invisible Friend gives me a nudge to assure me;
He is with me every moment of every day.

Since I've been redeemed, I've made many a friend,
Of which there seems to be no end.
But the one who said, "There is a friend that sticketh,
Closer than a brother," he is my Invisible Friend.

Now I know whatsoever battle I may go through,
I can have peace and joy unspeakable.
For my Invisible Friend, the Great Three in One,
Is "… a very present help in trouble."

Proverbs 18:24
Psalms 46:1

In his Word he tells us, "... I will never leave thee, nor forsake thee" (Hebrews 13:5). I cannot praise him enough for the salvation I received that blessed day thirty-eight years ago. He has been so faithful and precious to me since that day, and I am grateful every day for his unconditional love and finished work on Calvary. "Thanks be unto God for his unspeakable gift" (2 Corinthians 9:15).

We are so unworthy of this great gift of salvation. Yes, it is a gift! "For by grace are ye saved through faith; and that not of yourselves: it is the gift of God: not of works, lest any man should boast" (Ephesians 2:8–9). This is God's plan, so when we get to heaven, we cannot boast about what we did to work our way there. When we arrive at our eternal resting place, we will kneel before him in praise and adoration for his sacrificial death on the cross that provided the way for us. "... and so shall we ever be with the Lord" (1 Thessalonians 4:17).

Some of the final words of Jesus before his death were, "... It is finished ..." (John 19:30). There is nothing to be added to it. Then, on the third day, Jesus rose from the grave to become our living Savior. After a brief time upon the earth, he ascended into heaven and is sitting on the right hand of God, being an intercessor for us. It is all about Jesus, the Lamb of God, sacrificing his life for our sin and redemption. "Not by works of righteousness which we have done, but according to his mercy he saved us ..." (Titus 3:5). Works follow salvation to express our love for him and to serve him until he calls us home. "For if Abraham were justified by works, he hath whereof to glory; but not before God. For what saith the scripture? Abraham believed God, and it was counted unto him for righteousness" (Romans 4:2–3).

We cannot fully comprehend this great love of our Savior towards us. "And to know the love of Christ, which passeth knowledge, that ye might be filled with all the fulness of God" (Ephesians 3:19). God created man to fellowship with him, but because of Adam's sin of eating the fruit from the forbidden tree, the tree of the knowledge of good and evil, that fellowship was broken for all mankind. Sin originated when Adam disobeyed God, and the sinful nature passed upon everyone. We are born with the sinful nature. The only way to restore the fellowship is by accepting the finished work of Christ on Calvary for our sin. "Wherefore, as by one man sin entered into the world, and death by sin; and so death passed upon all men, for that all have sinned" (Romans 5:12). "For as in Adam all die, even so in Christ shall all be made alive" (1 Corinthians 15:22). It is only when we come to the knowledge that we were born sinners, with the Adamic nature, and believe that Jesus died for our sin and accept him as our Savior can we be saved and born again. Having the assurance of my salvation and knowing I had become a child of God, I knew whatever came into my life was for a purpose. No matter what comes my way, I will trust in him.

> For all have sinned, and come short of the glory of God.
> Romans 3:23
> But God commendeth his love toward us, in that,
> while we were yet sinners, Christ died for us.
> Romans 5:8

For the wages of sin is death; but the gift of God is eternal life through Jesus Christ our Lord.

Romans 6:23

That if thou shalt confess with thy mouth the Lord Jesus, and shalt believe in thine heart that God hath raised him from the dead, thou shalt be saved. For with the heart man believeth unto righteousness; and with the mouth confession is made unto salvation.

Romans 10:9–10

For whosoever shall call upon the name of the Lord shall be saved.

Romans 10:13

Ed and I returned the next week for the results of the PET scan. This report read negative as far as any other cancer being found elsewhere, only that in my breast. Praise the Lord! At this visit Dr. Mattison talked with us about my options. He explained the two types of surgery, which are a mastectomy or a lumpectomy. He suggested that we not make a sudden decision but go home and talk about it and return in one week.

Ed asked, "What would your recommendation be if this happened to your wife?"

He replied without hesitation, "I would recommend a lumpectomy, but if you asked my wife, she would have a mastectomy."

From the depths of my mind came this thought: *Lots of great help that is!*

I came home from that appointment and immediately started searching the Internet for answers. I found a site

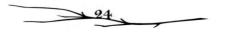

where an oncologist welcomed questions. I e-mailed her several times and received very informative, helpful, and mind-settling answers. When you are sitting in the doctor's office and receive such a troubling report, you cannot think of questions to ask at that moment. On your way home you think, *I wish I had thought to ask him this or this.* Dr. Mattison's nurse had given me several booklets to read on my first visit that were very informative. Through e-mails I had time to form in my mind questions to ask while in the confines of my home. I had given her the information in my reports so she could read them and base her answers on the reports. She was my second opinion, and I was confident when we made our decision it was the right one.

Alice Fletcher

Listen to God

Our almighty, omniscient God has the most
    powerful things to say;
It is from his holy Word that we receive guidance
    for every day.
In this world of fast pace, stopping and listening
    to him is a must,
For by his instructions is the only way to run
    the race set before us.

He speaks to us through preachers, teachers,
    and the written Word;
We must be quiet so we can ponder all the things
    we have heard.
Reading and heeding the Bible daily is but
    a small show of our love;
He is ever present and watches over us
    from his heavenly home above.

Through his Word he teaches us all things on
    how to live our life;
If we take heed to what he says, it will keep us
    from a world of strife.
When we are in our deepest despair and feel
    we have nowhere to go,
He sends comfort by the Holy Spirit,
    his everlasting love to show.

He yearns to communicate with us by feasting
    on his word each day,
Responding by prayer of praise and supplication

to what he has to say.
If we do not listen and obey him, we will not
    have the power to stand,
While Satan comes with his fiery darts as we
    walk this pilgrim land.

Therefore, listening and obeying God is the most
    important thing to do;
We can finish the race with joy and the trials of life
    may become few.
Because our Father will honor our loyalty through
    his sacrificial Son,
In heaven we can triumph because only by him was
    our race won.

Through My Valley

Ed and I prayed and discussed it many times during that week before my return visit. With further discussion with Dr. Mattison, I decided to have a lumpectomy.

My maternal grandmother had breast cancer back in the fifties and had one breast removed. That was the only procedure back then. I am so thankful for the advancements today for breast cancer surgery.

The surgery was scheduled for November 30, 2005.

The Sunday before my surgery, my Sunday school teacher at that time, Ray Turner, used the verse, "For God hath not given us the spirit of fear; but of power, and of love, and of a sound mind" (2 Timothy 1:7). In my heart I said, *Thank you, Lord. You gave that to him just for me.* I had not experienced anxiety yet, and this was telling me there is no need for fear. Since God does not give us a spirit of fear, fear must come from Satan.

During my surgery, not only was the cancer mass and surrounding tissue removed, but three lymph nodes leading out to my arm were removed. The doctor examined the nodes while I was still under anesthetic to see if the cancer had spread into the lymph nodes. If so, additional lymph nodes would have to be removed. Cancer cells were found in the first lymph node. They were floating cells and had not attached; therefore, additional nodes did not have to be removed.

My name was placed on our church prayer list, and as our friends heard of my cancer, they called to tell us they were praying for us and had placed my name on their churches' prayer lists. That week our daughter-in-law Alisia asked a fellow worker of hers, also a friend of ours who is a pastor's wife, to pray for me. Marianne told her I would be added to their prayer list.

Marianne and her family attended the same church we did some twenty-five years prior. The Lord had led us to another church, and Don, Marianne's husband, answered the call to the ministry, so our paths were parted. After Don graduated from Bible college, he was called to pastor a church in a town close to where we lived. We then regained our friendship, although we did not see each other often.

Marianne phoned to tell me she was praying for me and asked for the name of my doctor, as she had not had a mammogram in several years and had found a lump in her breast.

She called Dr. Mattison's office and made an appointment for the following week.

The pathology report came back from my surgery, also stating that the cancer did not originate in my breast. Therefore, Dr. Mattison had the specimen and reports sent to Vanderbilt University for further examination. The report came back stating the cancer was confined to the breast but should be regarded as an aggressive high-grade carcinoma, named Infiltrating Ductal Carcinoma, Stage Two.

I needed an additional surgery to remove more tissue from the area where the cancer was removed. A smaller tumor that was hidden by the tumor seen on the mammogram was found by the pathologist. This tumor was lying close to the edge of the flesh that was previously removed. When a cancer tumor is removed, not only the tumor but some flesh around it is removed. Upon finding the second tumor, Dr. Mattison felt more flesh had to be removed.

Dr. Mattison told me not to be surprised that I might need chemotherapy, based on the report from Vanderbilt University. He had previously told us that I might not need chemotherapy. I discussed with him that it was time for my five-year colonoscopy. This was mid-December, and I was due for the procedure in February. I definitely needed to have this done because of the history of colon cancer in my family. Three aunts, my mother's sisters, had passed away from colon cancer. I had this done religiously every five years. He informed me that chemotherapy causes the linings in the body to become thinner; therefore, he wanted me to have the colonoscopy before beginning chemotherapy, if I was to have the treatments. Receiving chemotherapy is determined by an oncologist. The colonoscopy was done on December 16 by my gastroenterologist, Dr. Woods. I made an appointment with him on the fourteenth, and, after hearing my situation, his office worked me in on the sixteenth for the procedure.

You are probably questioning, why get a colonoscopy when the PET scan showed there was no other cancer in my body? Polyps grow in the colon that later turn to cancer if they are not removed. Polyps do not show on the PET scan. I had had polyps removed previously, but this time the colonoscopy showed none.

On the day of my second surgery, December 21, Marianne received her report that she also had breast cancer. I knew her appointment was before my surgery.

After my surgery, I said, "Dr. Mattison, I don't imagine you will be able to tell me about Marianne's findings."

He replied, "Marianne told me I could tell you that she has cancer also."

After much prayer and searching the Internet, she also made the decision to have a lumpectomy.

Her surgery was one week later. Cancer was discovered in three lymph nodes; therefore, she had to have the remaining lymph nodes removed in her arm. Dr. Mattison told her the day of her surgery that she needed to make an appointment with an oncologist, based on having had the additional lymph nodes removed.

The week following my second surgery, I returned for a follow-up visit with Dr. Mattison. He made an appointment for me to see an oncologist the next week. I carried my records and X-rays to the oncologist's office prior to my appointment for the doctor to study. This appointment brought more dreaded news. Dr. York informed me I needed chemotherapy as well as radiation.

After my consultation with Dr. York, a nurse came and spent much needed time with Ed and me explaining what to expect from chemotherapy. The nurse told me my emotions might be on a roller-coaster ride, some dos and don'ts, and gave me three prescriptions for nausea. She explained how my white blood count would be low and I would be susceptible to colds and viruses, advising me not to get in crowds. She told us the treatments given in the arm could cause my veins to collapse; therefore, she recommended I get a port placed in my chest to receive the chemotherapy. The port would also be used to draw blood each visit to test my blood counts. Having the port would be my decision. Then she dropped the bomb—she told me I would lose my hair in approximately eighteen days after the first treatment.

The next week Marianne was given the same dreaded news by Dr. York.

At that time we became true bosom buddies.

I told many friends and e-mailed others that I had read of one breast cancer patient who had friends that shaved their heads with her. Did I have any takers?

I had no takers! I retract that statement. My brother, Don, told me he was going to have his head shaved if I was able to visit him during that time. Everyone knew I was just kidding anyway, because they all knew I already had someone committed to this, Marianne. Maybe I should not use the word committed because neither Marianne nor I willfully offered to do this.

Don was living in Blacksburg, Virginia. I was living in Molena, Georgia. Knowing he could not be close by me during my treatments, Don wanted to have a part in my procedures. He sent me a check for me to buy my wig and hats and to help on gas money traveling back and forth for treatments. The oncologist's office was forty miles away. This was a tremendous blessing to me! I shall never forget this kindness from his heart to me.

Due to the history of heart disease in my family and my ripe old age of sixty-six, Dr. York wanted me to have a MUGA scan before I started my treatments. A MUGA scan is done by injecting a radiation tracker into a vein and waiting thirty minutes for the tracker to tap onto blood cells and circulate in the chambers of the heart, after which an EKG is done to determine if the heart is strong enough to receive the chemotherapy treatments.

Marianne only needed a regular EKG before her treatments began, which she had the same day that I had my scan. After she finished her EKG, she and Don came to where Ed and I were.

When the technician called my name, Marianne asked if she could go with me. Of course he said yes. Ed and Don remained in the waiting room. This appointment took over an hour, including the time I waited for the tracker to circulate through my heart. During the scan we were talking with the technician about us both having breast cancer.

Somewhere in the conversation I said, "In a few short weeks we will be headless."

Marianne corrected me, "Alice, we will be hairless."

The technician immediately replied, "I could picture the two of you walking down the street without a head on your shoulders."

This broke Marianne and me up into hard laughter.

All of a sudden the technician yelled, "What's going on?"

He was looking at the monitor and it was going haywire. I had laughed so hard that three suction cups had become detached. He calmed us down so he could reattach the cups and continue with the scan.

This report gave me the okay to go ahead with chemotherapy treatments.

After our heart scans, we ate lunch together with our husbands, after which we went our separate ways to shop for wigs. An occasion that one would guess should have been a discouraging day turned out to be a fun day. The American Cancer Society had an office in the area where we were to get treatments. They offered two free wigs to cancer patients. We laughed and laughed as we tried on wigs. Knowing we would not stray too far from our natural color, brunette, didn't stop us from trying on many colors and shades, long, short, straight, and curly.

Even though we had not lost our hair yet, we each wore one wig home. I couldn't wait to arrive home to show Ed. He liked the wigs I picked out but found one in a catalog he liked much better, so I ordered it.

Alice Fletcher

Marianne and I both chose to have a port surgically implanted. We had this procedure done on the same day, at the same hospital, as outpatients, one right after the other.

I know that right about now you are thinking, *This woman is like The Rock of Gibraltar*. Oh, so far from the truth. The day of my port surgery, I completely lost it. Ed had a job that day that would last only a short time. Instead of him giving up this job or having it rescheduled, he took me to the hospital about forty-five minutes early, and our son Clint was coming to sit with me until Ed returned. I was filled to the brim with anxiety that day. After a biopsy, a PET scan, two surgeries, a colonoscopy, a visit with my oncologist, and a MUGA scan, this was going to be the seventh procedure in nine weeks. I was sitting by myself waiting for Clint to arrive and could feel the tears coming.

My oncologist's office was in the hospital complex, so I took off to talk with a nurse. Seated in the waiting room, waiting for her to call my name, I could hardly contain myself. The minute she called my name, the tears started rolling big time. I couldn't even get the words out of my mouth to let the nurse know what I was there for. The minute she looked at me she knew! She took me to an examining room, or I should say into a bawl room, and was extremely compassionate with me as I let it all out. She told me this was what I needed to do.

This was the first time I had cried over this journey through my valley. She gave me a complimentary anxiety pill and had the doctor write a prescription for the same, telling me I needed to have it filled and take one prior to each treatment.

I recovered and went back to meet Clint, trying to act as

if nothing had happened. Sometime later I told Clint this, and he said he knew. We are not very good at hiding these moments. My faith does not falter at these times. It just proves that we are still embodied in this body of flesh.

Then came the day, Tuesday, January 24, 2006, when Marianne and I began our first chemotherapy treatments. We were scheduled for treatments every two weeks. Marianne and I always scheduled our treatments on the same day, fifteen minutes apart, so we would be there for each other. We were both uptight that day not knowing the complete ramifications that would come from the treatment.

One thing I detest is being nauseated. I wondered if I would become nauseated during the treatments. Our son Mike, a survivor of Hodgkin's Lymphoma, told us of one time when he had gotten so sick in the middle of taking one treatment and how one time on the way home from treatments he had to pull over to the side of the road to throw up. The type of chemotherapy he received was a different type than I received. I was just sitting there waiting for it to come. Thankfully I got through it fine. In fact, that day was like any other, with absolutely no reaction from the treatment. Yet!

Most of our treatments lasted four hours, except the first treatment of Taxol, which we received during the second eight-week period of treatments. Taxol has to be administered slowly the first time because of potential bad side effects. This treatment took six hours to receive.

Many days between appointments Marianne and I would talk on the phone comparing our side effects.

Alice Fletcher

I praise the Lord for the knowledge he has given to the medical field. Although the first types of chemotherapy administered to us were very harsh, with the nausea medication I was spared being nauseated from these first treatments. Marianne did have some nausea after the first treatment. She called on Thursday to say she was sick and could not eat and to ask if I was sick as well. Her husband had gone to their church for church visitation and she was alone. I had cooked a large pot of chicken and rice soup prior to starting chemotherapy and had it in the freezer in individual freezer bags in case I got sick. Ed and I took her a container of the soup. She realized on the day of our first treatment she had forgotten to take the nausea-preventing medication we were to take one hour before the treatment was to begin. Needless to say, she never forgot again.

Even though I was not nauseated, I had to take the medication so I could eat because my appetite was nil. Although the medication helped, I could only eat very little at each sitting.

Right on schedule, on the seventeenth day after my first treatment, as I was brushing my hair that morning, a handful of hair came out. I went to art class that day, and upon returning I brushed my hair again and another handful came out. I must say, that was not an enjoyable experience.

That afternoon Ed and I went out on the porch for him to shave my head. I wanted him to do this rather than wake up one morning with hair all over my pillow.

We have a golden retriever named Buckshot, Buck for short, who came and put his head in my lap the entire time

Out of my Valley

Ed was shaving my head. With hair falling on him, he looked up with such sad eyes as if to ask, *What is going on?*

With four sons, Ed had a lot of experience cutting hair when they were growing up. There is scarcely a time when our four sons get together that the subject of hair cutting doesn't come up. One Christmas, Luke, our youngest son, gave Ed a gag gift, a video cassette titled *How to Cut Hair*. All four of our sons were in R.O.T.C. It occurred to me that maybe it was their way of finally having the opportunity to go to the barbershop.

Now came the time to start wearing my wig. I felt very comfortable and enjoyed wearing it.

I received many compliments. A lady at church came up to me and told me how well she liked the way I had my hair fixed. When I told her it was a wig, she acted shocked. I had several turbans I wore while in the house and several hats made for when I went out grocery shopping or riding around, when I felt up to it. Therefore, I gave one of the wigs I received from the cancer society to another patient and returned the other to the society for someone else to enjoy. The one I bought with the money Don gave me, I told him he could wear when we got together again, because he called it *our wig*.

I never realized how much warmth hair supplies. This was early February, and the turbans were a treasure to me. I even had a night cap I wore to bed because my bare head was cold.

Chemotherapy has a lot of side effects. It can change your taste, and it gives you a metal taste in your mouth. Canned fruit and celery were very refreshing to me. Most foods didn't taste the same. Anything sweet was magnified about four times and was impossible to eat. This was bad news for me, as I am a sweets eater. But praise the Lord, I found out I can live without all the sweets. I do not eat sweets as I used to.

One day Ed and I were gone from the house for a few hours, and upon returning we found a container of celery that a neighbor, Joyce, had left for me on our back porch. I had mentioned to her that celery was one thing I could eat and enjoy. I have always called Joyce the mother hen of our neighborhood, as she has that care-giving, nurturing gift. She is forever checking on neighbors.

Marianne and I would compare what we could and could not eat. Knowing I loved sweets, Marianne would call and say she bought a particular brand of fudge bars, so I would buy the same the next time I was in a grocery store. After one bite I found I could not tolerate them.

Later she would call and say, "Alice, I found the yummiest ice cream sandwiches." So, I purchased them to no avail. In reverse, there were things I could eat with no problem but she couldn't. Another person may have completely different side effects, although most are experienced by everyone.

The nursing staff had advised us to purchase and drink vitamin-filled shakes for strength and nutrition, since we didn't feel up to eating. Since I was not cooking and had zero appetite, I was not opening the refrigerator to see them, so I would forget, but my nursemaid, Ed, would remind me.

The first four treatments were the toughest. We were given two different kinds of chemotherapy simultaneously for these first treatments. These two were Adriamycin and

Cytoxan. They were administered every other week. The first two or three days after treatment, I was fine. Then for six to seven days, I was completely wiped out.

Our chemotherapy was received in liquid form through the port by IV. I have heard of oral and implanted seeds as treatment for other types of cancer also.

It caused me to be extremely weak and washed out. I could not stand up but for a short period of time. In the mornings I would get out of bed, go to the bathroom, then have to go back to bed to regain strength, get back up, go to the bathroom to wash up, go back to bed for a few minutes or so, get back up, and go brush my teeth.

I didn't have enough strength to stand long enough to cook a meal. I tried sitting on a stool to cook breakfast one Sunday morning and couldn't finish. I just slid the pan off the burner and went back to bed. After Ed got ready for church, he had to finish fixing breakfast. From then on he would tell me not to get up and fix breakfast. He would prepare breakfast even on the Sundays when I was able to attend church. I had always fixed a big breakfast on Sunday morning since we had been married.

I would take a stool with me into the shower to sit on, and being so tired after the shower, I didn't have the strength to dry off; my arms felt so heavy. After sitting a few minutes, I regained enough strength to finish the task at hand.

Then three to four days before my next treatment, I would revive and get some strength back, although not enough to be able to maintain the household. Around the time of my third treatment, I felt I was no longer able to drive safely for myself. Everywhere I went, Ed was my chauffeur. Therefore,

I had to put paint class on hold. It was another forty miles in another direction to class. Ed needed to go in that direction one Thursday, my scheduled day for class, so I decided to go to class while he did his running around. By the time we traveled there, I was too weak and shaky to stay for class. This thought came to me: *This too shall pass.*

Toward the end of the first eight weeks, I remember lying in bed (which was about all I could do), and Satan whispered to me one day, "How content are you now, big girl?"

Again, due to God's faithfulness, a verse that I had hidden in my heart was brought forth. You will read in God's Word, "For I reckon that the sufferings of this present time are not worthy to be compared with the glory which shall be revealed in us" (Romans 8:18).

I said to him, "Get thee behind me, Satan," and reminded him of his fate and that he would not be in heaven with us. He is the great deceiver and the deliverer of discouragement to us, if we yield to him instead of the Holy Spirit.

One day as I was just lying around thinking of my faith and remembering stories from the Bible, I began to think about the woman who had an issue of blood for twelve years, in Luke 8:43–48, and about her faith, knowing that all she had to do was reach out and touch the hem of Jesus' garment and he would make her whole. This woman needed healing. Our first step in faith is for our salvation. As I dwelt on that and thought about the faith we need for all aspects of our life, the Lord began to bring words to me for another poem. I remembered hearing a sermon many years ago about how three times the words, "The just shall live by faith," were stated in the Bible: (1) faith for our salvation; (2) faith for our daily living; and (3) faith looking forward to reaching our heavenly home. These are the words the Lord gave me.

Alice Fletcher

Reach Out and Touch Him

*The Just Shall Live by Faith

There was a woman, in the days when Jesus walked
    upon this earth,
Who had an issue of blood for twelve years.
After spending all her living upon physicians,
    neither could be
Healed by any, no doubt she had wept a lot of tears.
She heard Jesus was coming her way and believed
    if she but
Touched his garment, she could obtain her goal.
When Jesus perceived that virtue had gone
    out of him, when
Confronting her, he said,
    "Thy faith hath made thee whole."

Just like this woman, the impurities of our
    sinful life can only
Be healed when we reach out to Jesus
    as he passes by.
His holy Word tells us that we have to come
    to him by faith
To be cleansed and receive salvation; then he
    will surely satisfy.

Through studying his Word, our faith will increase,
    and as we
Put on the whole armor of God, we receive
    the power to stand.
He will guide our feet into the path of peace,

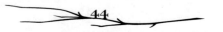

Out of my Valley

as we trust and obey
Him while on our journey through
    this pilgrim land.

As our days on this earth grow shorter,
    we marvel at God's love,
Mercy, and forgiveness towards us by his grace.
We know by faith that whether being
    raised from the grave or
Caught up to meet him in the air we
    shall fellowship with him
Throughout eternity face to face.

Romans 1:17—Salvation through faith
Galatians 3:11—Living by faith
Hebrews 10:36–39—Receive our
    eternal glory in faith

Onward Through My Valley

Having completed the first round of chemotherapy, we started on the next round, named Taxol, without a break in between. This was administered every two weeks as well for a total of eight weeks. This was still a pretty potent treatment but slightly better on the body, as far as weakness, than the first two. Although I was spared from nausea from the first treatments, I did get nauseated after each of these treatments on the second day and had to take medication for that one day.

The third day after each treatment of Taxol, I would have extreme pain in my bones so bad it would bring tears to my eyes. It was not joint pain but actually in the bones, in my lower spine and across my hips. The pain would not last long, maybe a few hours for one day. It was so severe I didn't want to move. As long as I lay completely still, I felt no pain. Nothing would relieve the pain, so my only choice was to remain still. I dreaded that time on Taxol. The nursing team in the oncologist's office was great about informing me of side effects. If they had not forewarned me of this, it would have scared the pudding out of me because it was so intense and came on suddenly without warning.

During this time, I developed suspected pneumonia. This made the Taxol treatments worse on me than they normally would have been. I had gotten weaker than usual and had difficulty breathing. I called the doctor's office and they asked me to come in. The office was on the fifth floor, and I told the nurse I didn't think I could make it up to the office, hardly being able to walk to the bathroom and back to bed. She told me there were wheelchairs at the hospital entrance. My husband drove me as close to the door as he could get to let me out, parked the car, and returned to wheel me to the doctor's office.

The doctor on duty that day saw in my chart that I am allergic to many things. He advised me to see my allergist. He called the respiratory department in the hospital for a nurse to come over to give me a breathing treatment, which helped me tremendously. Following the doctor's advice, I made an appointment to see my allergist and there was told I had suspected pneumonia. After a round of antibiotics and more bed rest, I recovered rather quickly.

I reflect back on that time when I was at my lowest physically. Ed came into the bedroom, and I told him he could take the money I had been saving for a newer car at the time of my retirement and put me in a nursing home. I was one miserable person during the time I had suspected pneumonia and was probably in a state of discouragement or depression, but we don't like to admit that. A few days later, after beginning to feel better, I remembered what I had said to Ed and felt terrible because of the TLC he was giving me, knowing he gave me far superior care than I would have received elsewhere.

During the second phase of my treatment, I began to regain some of my strength. I didn't have to take as much of the medications as before but still got tired quickly when I tried to do any household chores.

Not only did we lose all the hair on our heads but over most of our bodies. I didn't have to shave my legs or underarms any longer. Marianne and I lost almost all of our eyebrows and eyelashes before the last treatment of Taxol was given. After the last treatment, our hair started growing back slowly. Our last treatment was May 2, 2006, but it was mid-November before my hair was long enough that I felt comfortable not wearing my hats or wig. One day I was with a friend and she picked a fallen hair off of my shoulder.

I said to her, "One would usually say, 'Oh no, I'm losing my hair!' But not me; I say praise the Lord! I have hair to lose."

I had straight hair before and was hoping for it to come back with a little curl. I was not fortunate for that to happen. I had thick hair before, but it came back thin as baby hair and remains that way today.

My hair is so soft that my granddaughter Taylor, upon feeling it for the first time, said, "Granny, your hair feels like a baby chicken."

I also lost a toenail during the treatments, and two fingernails detached from the skin underneath, as if I was going to lose them also. I did not lose the fingernails, but it took months for them to reattach as the nails grew out. We also developed neuropathy in our feet and fingers. This numbness is due to restricted circulation. Dr. York informed me that this was temporary in a vast majority of cases but has been known to become permanent for some patients. Mine has begun to subside some to the point it is not as bothersome to me now. If it becomes permanent at this stage, it will be bearable. I have always loved to go barefoot, but it feels like needles sticking in my feet if I do go barefoot now.

When I think of pain in my body, it is not long before I am reminded of the pain Christ suffered for me when he willingly went to the cross for me. There is nothing in me compared to the agony he went through as he was spat upon, his beard ripped from his face, beaten beyond recognition, and a crown of thorns placed on his head; I can only imagine it was not placed there very gently. In shame and humility he carried his heavy cross to his ultimate death, as spikes were driven through his hands and feet as he was nailed to that old rugged cross. As he cried, "I thirst," he was given vinegar to drink as the bystanders laughed and mocked him. Then, finally the sins of the whole world were poured out on him as God himself could not look upon him. Darkness fell upon the world for three hours as this was accomplished, while Jesus cried out, "My God, My God, why hast Thou forsaken me?" (Matthew 28, Mark 15).

Another side effect is called chemo brain. It is manifested by forgetfulness. One can be in the middle of a sentence and completely forget what they are saying. One day I heard Ed talking on the telephone with one of our sons explaining this to him. Clint had noticed this in my speech and was concerned that I might be getting dementia or Alzheimer's. Subsequently he had called Ed to talk with him about this. I keep blaming this on the treatments, but lately I am having too many people jokingly (I hope) tell me I had this problem way before chemotherapy.

Ed became a tremendous housekeeper and nursemaid. I let everyone know after I got back on my feet again I was going to hire him out, but I was going to milk it to the end. In reality, I couldn't wait to get back to doing household chores and cooking again.

His dedication and devotion to me during this time brought to mind the scripture, "Husbands, love your wives, even as Christ also loved the church, and gave himself for it" (Ephesians 5:25). Ed completely gave of himself to serve me during this time. Not only was my Lord with me, but Ed was also there every step of the way—each doctor's visit, each treatment, and simple words of encouragement along the way.

He did cooking and cleaning up after. Until this time I didn't know he knew how to turn the vacuum cleaner on, but he did a wonderful job, and hold on, ladies—he even scoured the bathroom sink, shower, and toilet to meet health department standards! I don't believe he dusted. We came from dust and shall return to dust, so maybe he thought he would disturb someone.

Alice Fletcher

Why Dust?

Okay! Go on and dust every week if you just have to,
But there are more exciting things in this life to do.
Like going to the dentist, or having a pap smear,
Men, as you wait as your prostate exam draws near.

Walking the dog in the pouring down rain,
Doing such things people will think you insane.
Life is so short; the older you get how quickly time flies.
Enjoy every moment. Don't waste them on
    jobs you despise.

What is a little allergic reaction,
    runny nose and itchy eyes,
Although there are some who will say this is not wise.
As you can see the one chore I hate is to dust,
But there are those of you that consider it a must.

"For dust thou art, and unto dust shalt thou return."
Dusting may disturb someone, causing others concern.
Dust if you wish, if that is what you do;
Just remember one day the dust may be you!

Genesis 3:19

Out of my Valley

Ed is a retired letter-carrier with the post office and now works part time doing inspection work. Many of his jobs only last a few hours. One particular day he had to be gone from the house many hours. Not knowing at the time that his concern for me being alone was so great, he called a neighbor, unbeknownst to me, and asked if she would come sit with me a while that day.

Mary was a dedicated walker and passed our house on her daily walk; sometimes she stopped in for a chat. On this particular day she came up the driveway and sat and talked for a longer spell than usual. When Ed arrived home, he inquired if Mary had come by, and I realized then he had called Mary to ask her to stop by and check on me. Mary and her husband, Harold, have moved away from the neighborhood now and are greatly missed.

During the weeks of treatments I lost twenty pounds, pounds of which I could easily spare. In December of each year, between Christmas and New Year's, my brother, Don, and his wife, Jan, come to visit. Every year, for years without fail, we talk about which one will lose the most weight before we see each other again in July, when Ed and I travel to Virginia to visit them. Each time I talked with Don by phone I would mention I was losing weight.

Toward the end, right before my last treatment of Taxol, I was talking with him and said, "I am beginning to get some strength back and feeling better. I have already lost twenty pounds."

He replied, "I have been waiting for you to say you are getting better and on your way to recovery because I have wanted to tell you this; you would do anything to win a bet."

I still didn't "win the bet" (no money involved). He had started going to a fitness center and cut back on his eating and had lost thirty-six pounds, which was more than Jan and I combined had lost.

All during our treatments, Marianne and I would count the weeks down until our final treatment. We could not wait for the last treatment to be over with. The day for my last treatment of Taxol, I could feel anxiety arising in me. The thought came to me: *Have I had enough of this harsh chemotherapy to eradicate this monster of cancer out of my body?* I knew the next round of chemotherapy was going to be mild in comparison to what we had been receiving. I talked with the nurse about my feelings on that day, and she told me many people have the same concerns. On that day, May 2, 2006, I was started on the last phase of chemotherapy treatments, named Herceptin. Marianne had to receive this also.

Herceptin travels through the body and attacks any cancer cells floating around and kills them. This is administered through the port as well. We received this every third week for one year. It is very mild and only caused me slight tiredness for a few days, and sometimes a decrease in my appetite, not enough that I was still losing weight. I began to regain more strength and some of the weight I had lost.

Herceptin has many side effects listed in the medical books, about two and a half columns, from low energy up to congestive heart failure. People would ask me the side effects since I was doing so much better on Herceptin.

My reply always was, "Not much, just congestive heart failure."

Inevitably everyone would say, "Oh! Is that all?"

Out of my Valley

I don't mean to make jest of this, but an extremely high majority of patients experience only low energy. The medical books have to list every side effect that might be a possibility. Marianne did experience laryngitis between each treatment. Her voice would get better before the next treatment, and a few days after the treatment she had problems again. Another disturbing side effect both Marianne and I experienced from all four types of chemotherapy was restless sleep, waking up every two hours just like clockwork, and crazy dreams, I mean *crazy* dreams. It would be some time before getting back to sleep. This just added to our tiredness.

Summer was on the horizon, garden planting time. We have always had a large vegetable garden. Ed decided not to plant such a large one because I might not have my strength built up enough to stand the many hours it takes. Some days in years gone by, it had been an all-day process. When the vegetables were ready to pick, I had to put everything else aside and prepare and process them for canning and freezing. He did plant a small garden, enough for us to eat from. The Lord had given us a bountiful crop the year before, and I had preserved enough to carry us through two winters. Another promise from the Lord, "But my God shall supply all your need according to his riches in glory by Christ Jesus" (Philippines 4:19).

My family and many friends showered me with get-well cards and telephone calls. Most calls Ed had to handle. Our four sons kept in touch, even though they had such busy lives with work and family. What an overwhelming joy to hear each of our sons tell me they were praying for me.

My daughter-in-law Kacey would send me the sweetest cards every few weeks, as did many friends and others from my church. I didn't feel up to using my computer much during those low times, but on the days I did, I would have e-mails from my daughter-in-law Ginger and Kacey's mother, Patti Byrne, that were always encouraging and said each was praying for me. Alisia would call frequently to check on me.

Many weeks Todd and Stacy Free, fellow church members, had cut flowers sent to our home with the sweetest note to show us their love, concern, and prayers for us. Our pastor at the time, Dr. David McCoy, would call after every treatment to see how I was doing, pray over the phone with us, and let us know he was praying for us daily. We have some wonderful neighbors that brought us delicious meals during this time.

The Lord convicted me during this time that I had not been as compassionate to others as they had been to me. I vowed to be a better servant for him. Oh, how the Lord uses others to speak to our heart.

Even children can be a blessing. Several men in our church came to Ed and told him their families, including the children, were praying for us. I wasn't strong enough the week after treatment to attend church but could attend the second Sunday before my next treatment. Ed and I would sit in a far back corner of the church away from the majority of the people and leave immediately after the service to avoid close contact with others. Many fellow worshipers would look back at me and mouth to me, *I'm praying for you.*

Out of my Valley

One Sunday, I happened to look toward the pew where we normally sat. The pew in front of our pew was where the Free family always sat. Kevin, the ten-year-old son, saw me sitting in the back of the church, probably the first time he saw me since I started wearing my wig. He was talking with Carol Lee, his grandmother, and I could imagine their conversation, because his eyes got so big and I could read his lips when he said, "She lost all of her hair!" then glanced back at me. That tickled me so much. I still smile when I think about it.

On Easter Sunday, Kevin's older sister, Kelly, brought me a piece of paper on which Kevin had drawn a picture of Calvary, with the three crosses, and the word Easter written on it. Kevin, thinking of me and showing his concern in this small way, meant so much to me. I cherish that picture and will always keep it in my Bible. I have wondered if Kevin sent the picture to me by his sister because maybe he thought I was contagious and didn't want to get near me. Never diminish the thoughts and prayers from children that show they care about you.

There were some people who distanced themselves from me at this time but let it be known through others of their concern. I can fully understand, as I have been that way in the past. People deal with situations in their own way that might not be the same way you would handle the same situation. It did not bother me at all. I know in the past there have been times when I have distanced myself from a situation because I didn't know what to say or do. I do pray this will not be the case in the future for me. I need to seek the Lord to put the needed words in my mouth for someone at such a time, or sometimes just one's silent presence is all that is needed to show compassion and concern. I know when I am not feeling well I would rather have silence, as others have said they feel the same way. After Job's second encounter with Satan, his three friends came to him "… to mourn with him and to comfort him" (Job 2:11). "So they sat down with him upon the ground seven days and seven nights, and none spake a word unto him: for they saw that his grief was very great" (Job 2:13).

In mid-May my daughter-in-law Alisia phoned to ask if I would walk the Relay for Life with her. Her office was sponsoring a booth for the event. She is also a cancer survivor. She had a cancerous tumor in her lower arm when she was a teenager. It was removed with surgery and she was advised to have chemotherapy, but her mother refused.

Having just finished my most harsh treatments, I told her I would try to walk around the field one time with her, but what would happen if I couldn't make it all the way around? She told me there would be helpers with wheelchairs around the field to give aid to anyone that needed it. We arrived at the field along with many cancer survivors and a throng of supporters.

After an inspiring program, the announcement was made for only cancer survivors on the track to begin the walk. After we made one lap around the track, anyone could walk the Relay for Life with us. Oh, what an uplifting experience I received from the supporters that were lined around the field. Everyone was clapping for us as we walked that first lap. I had never experienced anything like it before. Drawing a boost of energy from all the support, I walked two laps. My eyes welled up with tears as I looked upon the mass of people looking on. I am looking forward to making that walk many more times in the coming years.

Now came the time for me to begin radiation treatments. Before my first radiation treatment, I went to the office to be tattooed. Small tattoos about the size of a head on a pin were tattooed on the outskirts of where the radiation was to be administered.

During the months of June and July 2006, I had radiation treatments every day, Monday through Friday, for six-and-a-half weeks, a total of thirty-three treatments. Needless to say, we didn't have the opportunity to visit Don and Jan that year, because I had my last treatment on Wednesday and school started the next Monday. Neither were we able to go on the week camping trip we had planned with two of our sons and their families. Although, we did have the opportunity to drive up to the camp site on Friday after my treatment to spend one night, get some trout fishing in, and enjoy the brief time with them.

The daily treatments take only a few minutes. Patients are scheduled for appointments fifteen minutes apart. The majority of the time in the treatment room was used to make sure the machine was lined up at the proper angle within the tattoos to zap me so the lungs and heart were not affected from the radiation. The actual zapping took minimal time. When the machine started, I would count one thousand one, one thousand two, etc., up to forty-five. Then the machine would turn to another angle and I would count the same until I reached twenty-eight, and it was over.

Alice Fletcher

The most aggravating part of the whole process was the fifty-mile roundtrip I had to drive each day. There is a penalty you must pay when you live in the boonies so far away from civilization, but the benefits of serene living far outweigh the penalty. We live so far out that if we are out of bread or milk, the nearest country store is six miles away (twelve miles roundtrip). For this reason I try to keep stocked up on groceries for the pantry and freezer.

One noticeable side effect from radiation is burning of the skin in the area of treatment. I applied a prescription cream twice a day to limit the intensity of the burning. My skin never did get badly burned, just extremely red. Some patients, men and women, get so badly burned that the treatments have to be stopped. The nurse told me people with fair skin were more susceptible to harsh burning. For our radiation treatments, Marianne and I chose different doctors, but we kept in touch frequently to compare treatment.

Another side effect is the forming of scar tissue. About six months after I had completed radiation, I had to go for rehabilitation therapy to learn how to massage the area to soften the scar tissue, as it was causing discomfort and had gotten painful for me to raise my arm. The therapist said there was scar tissue from my surgeries as well, mainly from the surgery in 1987.

Radiation treatments can only be administered one time in the same area. If I happen to have cancer reappear in my right breast, radiation will not be an option. I can receive treatments if cancer develops in my left breast or elsewhere, but prayerfully this will not happen.

With the three lymph nodes leading to my underarm

having to be removed from my right side when I had my initial surgery, my right arm cannot be used to take blood pressure, to have blood drawn for testing, or IVs inserted in the future. The rehabilitation therapist informed me I should use my right arm only for a brief time each time I am doing something, maybe fifteen or twenty minutes. This I forget, because if I am working outside pulling weeds, digging around in flowerbeds, or spending a good part of my day doing housework, I will end up with my lower arm and hand either with numbness or pain for several days. This is because the lymphatic fluids have been restricted from circulating after the nodes were removed. This is more of a problem for me than Marianne because I am right-handed. She also is right-handed, but her surgery was on her left side.

After the lymph nodes are removed, there is danger of developing lymphedema, a condition where excess fluid collects in tissue and causes permanent swelling in the arm. Receiving radiation treatments in that area may also be a cause. I pray this never happens to me.

The first day of the 2006–2007 school year began on August 1. I had been on sick leave from November 30, 2005, through the last day of the school year of 2005–2006. The Lord had blessed me with good health over the past years, and I had accumulated enough sick leave days to carry me through the time I was out, except for six days. I was a member of the sick leave bank and was able to retrieve the six days' pay from the bank. I had been donating one day a year from my sick leave to the bank for many years. Dr. York had informed me I should stay out of crowds and close quarters, and it was imperative that I not get in contact with anyone with chicken pox. A child is contagious with chicken pox before they break out. My treatments were in the height of chicken pox season, and with the close quarters on a school bus, he advised me to not work. With such weakness from the treatments, I can't imagine how I would have been able to drive a school bus safely anyhow.

I returned to work and was overjoyed to return. Two elementary schools were redistricted due to the opening of a new middle school. Quite a bit more was added to my route, in mileage as well as the number of students. It was hard on me to get up at 4:45 a.m. (earlier than years before), prepare myself to leave the house, drive the twenty-two miles to the bus shop to get my bus, do the bus inspection every morning, and drive fifteen more minutes to get out to the beginning of my route to start picking up students by 6:30 a.m. I asked for some relief to no avail.

I was talking to a fellow driver about the situation and said to her, "It is time to give this up after thirty-three years."

I was upset at first that this decision had to be made, as I had planned on driving at least two more years. One afternoon driving home this scripture came to me: "And we know that all things work together for good to them that love God, to them who are the called according to his purpose" (Romans 8:28). I knew this was God's way of telling me it was time to retire, and I must accept the decision with satisfaction. So, I submitted my retirement papers, and two weeks later, on August 31, 2006, I retired. I have enjoyed my retirement up to this point and have never looked back, believing this was God's will. I believe had I not been out on sick leave for the six months of the previous school year, I would have had a harder time with this adjustment in my life. I do miss the children and the precious things that have happened over the years. Children can say and do the cutest things without knowing. There were many exasperating moments over the years also. That is another book in itself.

Our son Clay and his wife, Kacey, called to break the news that she was pregnant. I don't know if they were any more excited than we were. It was their first child. This was around the last of September, and we traveled to Florida to visit them in October. This was the first long trip since I started treatments. The trip was very tiring, but it was such a blessing to be with them and see their excitement over the upcoming blessed event. Kacey is a schoolteacher, and they had planned for the baby to be due around the time school would be out for the summer. Her doctor calculated her due date to be the day after post-planning. You can't plan any closer than that.

But, much to everyone's sorrow, they telephoned us in late October to say the fetus had stopped growing. She had a D&C the first part of November. During the night after we got the telephone call about their misfortune, I awoke with this thought on my mind: *We never know what lies around the bend, but when a setback comes into our life, we need not be discouraged, as it is there to keep us from tragedy further down the road, and not be afraid when we approach the next bend in our life.* I got out of bed at 1:00 a.m., sat down in front of my computer, and started writing the following. Before I continue on, I do want to say with joy Clay called in February to say Kacey was pregnant again. I prayed that this bend in their road would bring them the most beautiful sight they have ever seen. October 26, 2007, a beautiful, healthy grandson was born. Aaron Bryant became our fifth biological grandchild; with three step-grandchildren, that brings the total to eight, ranging up to twenty-one years old.

Out of my Valley

Our Christian Journey

There are two roads in life. We are born on the highway of destruction, called the Broadway. As we begin our journey through this life, we must decide somewhere along the way to turn and get on the highway that leads to eternal rest. This highway is called the Strait-way. As we begin to travel this highway, bought by the shed blood of Jesus Christ, we must yield to the Holy Spirit, fall in close behind him, and follow after him the entire journey.

This journey will take us across lofty mountain heights, through deep valleys, and we will not always have sunshine. As we are going through that violent storm, we must remember the clouds will soon open up and the sun will come shining through again. Keep in mind he made the storms as well as the sunshine. Fret not, as he knows our every situation at all times.

As we see a crossroad ahead, we must seek his guidance before going in a new direction. If he doesn't turn to take a new direction, neither should we, but totally depend on his leadership.

Soon we come to a bend in the road. We must trust him to see us around it. There may be an obstacle in the road that causes us to have a setback. At this point we must pull over to restore it. We find he has not gone ahead but stayed with us to encourage us and support us. We give thanks for the obstacle, as it may have kept us from a tragedy further down the road. Continuing on, as we approach the next bend in the road, we should not hesitate to go around it, as we may behold the most beautiful sight that is far beyond our expectation.

Up ahead we see a fork in the road. He knows that one way is long and smooth, and the other way is short, bumpy, and risky. He chooses to go the long way; we choose the short way. We find it very dangerous and a lonesome trip without him leading us. We miss the closeness we had with him and regret that we chose to go our own way. Being of the omniscient Godhead, he knows both roads intersect. As we approach the intersection, we find him waiting for us. Although he took the long way, it was the quickest and most desirable way. Oh, how it brings joy as we realize we can be in fellowship with him anew as we repent and determine not to stray again from his guidance, as we continue on our journey until we reach our final destination.

Ultimately our heavenly home!

Matthew 7:13–14

Out of My
Valley

On April 24, 2007, fifteen months of chemotherapy treatments were completed, the last twelve months being Herceptin, which did not carry all the awful side effects as the other types.

On my first follow-up visit, Dr. York's joyous words to me were, "Alice, based on your blood work, everything looks great, and I am giving you a clean bill of health. You will have to return to the office periodically for blood work for the next three and a half years until your five-year anniversary of being cancer free is reached."

This is calculated from the date of surgery. I will not have to take a medication by mouth that some women do because I am ER negative.

Marianne, Don, Ed, and I spent many an hour in the

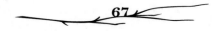

treatment room making up for all the years gone by. Every two weeks we had our fellowship time together. What a blessing to have someone with you during treatments. The time goes by so much faster. If there may be someone you know having to take treatments and no one else is able to be with them at the time because of work, other obligations, etc., what a great ministry it would be to accompany them to their treatments.

Two weeks after our last treatment, Marianne and I each had our port surgically removed as outpatient surgery, with the hope that one will never need to be inserted again.

Some of the side effects from the chemotherapy still remain. When carrying on a conversation, I still have a problem remembering names and objects in the middle of a sentence. This is very frustrating! Waking up many times during the night, having the crazy dreams, and the neuropathy are still with me. The medication to help me sleep soundly works and does stop the crazy dreams, but it can be addictive; therefore, I don't take it often. Back during the month of August, while I was still driving the school bus, to ensure a good night's sleep for safety purposes, I would take it, maybe twice a week. I have no idea how long this will last because Ed's sister and cousin still have these side effects after two years after finishing their chemotherapy treatments; although, they are both on the medication Tomaxifm.

On Thanksgiving Day 2007, after we had enjoyed a wonderful dinner with most of our family present, we went outside to throw the football around, which sometimes leads into an out and out football game with the younger adults and grandchildren.

As I threw the football to Brantley, our grandson, he yelled out, "Wow, Granny still has it!"

Growing up with three brothers, I became a pretty good football, baseball, and basketball player, and yes, I still have it. Well, some of it.

There are three reasons I titled this *Out of My Valley*. To share my experience and pray it will be helpful to others going through their valley, whatever their valley may be; to share the spiritual lessons I learned; and to show that faith in the Lord Jesus Christ can be a life full of joy at all times. The Lord blessed me tremendously as I walked through this deep valley through healing and through spiritual growth, thanks to the prayers of many.

Reason 1: The Lord has brought me *Out of My Valley* based on my blood test report that showed me to be cancer free. This is not a path I would have chosen to take. While in the valley, the Lord showed me that by his grace I was able to endure with joy because of his presence with me.

Reason 2: To share the spiritual lessons I gleaned from the *Out of My Valley* experience and show that our valleys can be a time of learning and blessing from the Lord as he strengthens and teaches us.

"The Lord on high is mightier than the noise of many waters, yea, than the mighty waves of the sea" (Psalm 93:4). Just think of the power and strength in these words. We do serve a mighty, powerful God. The God who spoke this vast universe into existence and created all things knows and cares for me. He is the great physician and has power to heal if it is his will.

In the midnight hour of our despair, God is not asleep.

During my treatments I heard a magnificent sermon on the storms in our life. I related it to my valley. Read Matthew 14:22–29. When Jesus sent his disciples out on the sea, he knew beforehand the storm was coming. God creates problems in our life. God puts us into storms to protect us from greater storms to come. God will put you into something to keep you out of something. People pray for things they are not ready for. God sends storms to develop and mature us, but we want the higher position without going through the storms. Jesus had to prove them. Jesus was walking on top of what they were afraid of, the raging sea. Jesus let them see him as they had never seen him before. Jesus is in the midst of the storm (valley) with you. Any storm (valley) is worth going through if you will see Jesus in it and mature spiritually from it.

After the midnight hour is the dawning of a new day.

"It is a good thing to give thanks unto the Lord, and to sing praises unto thy name, O most High: To shew forth thy lovingkindness in the morning, and thy faithfulness every night" (Psalm 92:1–2). No matter what you go through, it is for a purpose. You may not know the purpose at the beginning of your storm, valley, or trial, but sooner or later he will show you. The reason may be to make you a stronger Christian, a test of your faith, a testimony to strengthen another person, or even chastisement. He may get us down just for us to realize, "Be still, and know that I am God..." (Psalm 46:10). Sometimes God has to make us examine ourselves to see what we are made of and afterwards come to the realization we need to make some changes. Pray that the Lord will show you and use you for his glory, and sing praises to him for the lessons learned. We need to praise him always for his everlasting love, his kindness, and his faithfulness toward us.

During a sermon, my pastor used the scripture in Psalm 116. He preached on verse fifteen; however, verse twelve pierced my heart as he was reading the complete psalm. "What shall I render unto the Lord for all His benefits towards me?" (Psalm 116:12). Eternity will not be long enough to thank him for all he has done for me in the past, the present, and the future! There is absolutely no way to calculate all his benefits toward me. I must get on with the work for my Lord in my living and in my witness, although it will be impossible to render all that is due to him. We should give thanks to the Lord with our lips and our lives, praising him with our thanksgiving and our thanks-living. Four times in Psalm 107 it says, "Oh that men would praise the Lord for his goodness, and for his wonderful works to the children of men!"

I have known the following all my Christian life because the Lord has brought forth Bible verses I have memorized many times when I was talking with someone, in my moment of despair, or when I have been studying my Bible. During my time of complete silence, when I was so weak I could not read my Bible, couldn't watch television, and just wanted to lie still in bed, the Lord brought scriptures to me. His promise for this is, "But the Comforter, which is the Holy Ghost, whom the Father will send in my name, he shall teach you all things, and bring all things to your remembrance, whatsoever I have said unto you" (John 14:26).

"Notwithstanding the Lord stood with me, and strengthened me ..." (2 Timothy 4:17).

The Lord showed me through others how I should be more compassionate and involved in the lives of other people while they are going through difficult times.

God's grace is sufficient for anything you are going through. Grace for each and every need. "Let us therefore come boldly unto the throne of grace, that we may obtain mercy, and find grace to help in time of need" (Hebrews 4:16). That marvelous grace is there for the asking.

Reason 3: I have to share my testimony. The deepest valley the Lord brought me out of was my valley of sin and unbelief, thirty-eight years ago, on the day I accepted him as my Savior. I shall never forget that day. We always remember important dates in our life, such as graduation days, date of marriage, the birth dates of our children, etc. You can even remember the weather on those days. So, how can one not remember the day when they were transformed from death unto life as they received Jesus as their Savior? Satan tries to make you forget. You may not be able to tell the specific date, but you will remember the transformation that took place because of the change in your life. "Therefore if any man be in Christ, he is a new creature: old things are passed away; behold, all things are become new" (2 Corinthians 5:17).

As I tried to go to sleep on a Sunday night, the convicting power of the Holy Spirit came to me with the thought that if I died during the night I knew I would not go to heaven. I mentioned this to Ed, and when he went to work, he contacted Dan Harden and asked him to come to our home to talk with me. That Monday about 2:00 p.m., sitting in a rocking chair on our back porch in early July 1970, I humbly asked for forgiveness of my sins and asked Jesus to come into my life.

The day started out as a typical, hot, muggy, sunny Georgia summer day but turned into the most beautiful day of my life. The Scriptures say all things become new. The grass looks greener, the sky bluer, and even the bird's song is sweeter, but the greatest things were the love for the things of God. Pleasures of yesterday became things I did not want or need anymore. Jesus Christ filled the void I had been trying to fill with the pleasures of this old world.

Dan Harden sat for a while longer and showed me scriptures that helped my understanding about salvation, being eternally secure, the indwelling Holy Spirit, the promise of heaven, and God's everlasting love.

One need not be in church at the altar to be saved and born again. Ed was sitting in his mail delivery truck the day he received salvation through Jesus Christ. Dan had been quoting Scripture to him during the previous months. The convicting power of the Holy Spirit was so strong that day that he had to submit and pray a prayer of repentance.

The happiness I thought I knew before does not compare with the joy in my life now. "Therefore being justified by faith, we have peace with God through our Lord Jesus Christ" (Romans 5:1). Without the peace with God, there can be no true joy. We realize the joy we have comes from him because Jesus said, "Be of good cheer," several times in the Scriptures. "...be of good cheer; thy sins be forgiven thee" (Matthew 9:2). "…Be of good cheer; it is I; be not afraid" (Matthew 14:27, Mark 6:50). "…be of good cheer; I have overcome the world" (John 16:33). "Rejoice evermore" (1 Thessalonians 5:16). Not just in the good times. We can rejoice, be of good cheer, and have joy because we have forgiveness by him, companionship with him, and victory through him.

I thank the Lord for my valley, for I have learned so much traveling through it and have grown closer to him than ever before. I do not know what the future holds as far as the cancer returning, but he knows. Cancer is a very scary thing, but this one thing I know: if he chooses to take me out of this world, I will immediately be with him, or if I live on, he will be with me! What greater promise is there than this one? In the scope of eternity, we will be with him in just a moment of time anyway! I don't dwell on the possibility of cancer returning, but on the days I go for blood work, I get anxious feelings on the way to the doctor's office.

On one occasion as we were sitting in the waiting room, I was telling Marianne of my feelings, and she said, "You know, I have the same feelings."

Her husband looked at both of us with a surprised look.

I said, "I know, O ye of little faith."

As he started to speak, Marianne spoke up ahead of him saying, "Don't say a word until you have walked in our moccasins."

I dare say, no matter how strong a person is, there will be times of anxiety. It is at times like this that we realize exactly how weak we are and that our strength comes from our Lord alone, by him and through him.

Out of my Valley

My prayer is that everyone who reads this knows without a doubt that if something happened and they have a sudden, unexpected death or if they live to old age, they know where they will spend eternity. Upon God's Word there is only one of two places the soul will go upon death, either heaven or hell. I have the assurance that I will be with my Lord in heaven when I leave this world. God's Word tells us we can know for sure. "But these are written, that ye might believe that Jesus is the Christ, the Son of God; and that believing ye might have life through his name" (John 20:31).

> And this is the record, that God hath given to us eternal life, and this life is in his Son. He that hath the Son hath life, and he that hath not the Son of God hath not life. These things have I written unto you that believe on the name of the Son of God; that ye may know that ye have eternal life, and that ye may believe on the name of the Son of God.
>
> 1 John 5:11–13

The Bible teaches that there is only one sin that will send us to hell, that being the sin of unbelief. Almost everyone is familiar with John 3:16, but do you know the verses that follow?

> For God so loved the world, that he gave his only begotten Son, that whosoever believeth in him should not perish, but have everlasting life. For God sent not his Son into the world to condemn the world; but that the world through him might be saved. He that believeth on him is not condemned: but he that believeth not is condemned already, because he hath

not believed in the name of the only begotten Son of God.

John 3:16–18

What joy it brings to know that I have that everlasting life because I am a "whosoever." That word, "whosoever," means anyone and everyone.

Your first step to salvation is to realize you are a sinner, that you have the nature of Adam in you. It is not sin that produces the sinner but the sinner that produces the sin.

Second, acknowledge that you are a sinner and believe the purpose for Jesus being born of a virgin and coming down from glory to live among us was to die on the cross for your sin and that he was resurrected for your justification. The Bible tells us that the Virgin Mary miraculously conceived by the Holy Spirit; therefore, Jesus did not have the nature of Adam in him. He is the only sinless one.

Third, pray and believe Jesus died on the cross for you and arose from the dead and is sitting at the right hand of God being an intercessor for you.

Just knowing this is not enough. Many people know but have not personally repented and accepted Christ as their Savior. Is there a time in your life when you acknowledged to God that you are a sinner and you needed him? If you cannot remember a time such as this, today should be that day.

A Sample Prayer:

God, I know I am a sinner. I believe Jesus died on the cross for my sins and arose to be my living Savior. I ask you to come into my heart, forgive me of my sins, and save my soul. I accept you now as my Savior. In Jesus' name, I pray. Amen.

Many people think they have to stop being as they are before they can become a Christian. But it is God's power that changes you after you accept Jesus as your Savior. "… behold, now is the accepted time; behold, now is the day of salvation" (2 Corinthians 6:2). You come to him just as you are. He is waiting to change your life from darkness into his marvelous light. You will always have the Adam nature, but you will receive the Holy Spirit in you to guide and strengthen you to live for him, a meaningful life. You will never know such peace in your life until you accept him as Savior and depend on him to guide you. The world has always cried out, *peace, peace.* That empty place people try to fill through searching for worldly pleasures can only be filled with the peace that comes through Jesus Christ. Wars and conflicts will always be. There will be no earthly peace until the Prince of Peace returns in his glory, but we can have that individual peace. "And the peace of God, which passeth all understanding, shall keep your hearts and minds through Christ Jesus" (Philippians 4:7). "Therefore being justified by faith, we have peace with God through our Lord Jesus Christ" (Romans 5:1).

If you sincerely prayed this prayer in repentance, your next step is to start reading the Bible (I recommend the King James Version) and start attending a true Bible-believing church. You may be asking, "What church should I attend?" That is where prayer comes into your life. Ask the Lord to direct you to the right church as you ask him to open your eyes and heart to the reading and understanding of the Bible. It will amaze you as God starts answering your prayers and guiding you into his way.

Use discernment when you hear or read little sayings that may sound good. Many are not scripturally sound. Example: At one time this bumper sticker was on many cars: "God is my co-pilot!" As for me, I want God to be my pilot; I will take the co-pilot seat! I am reminded of a popular saying I first heard in the 70s, "God said it, I believe it, and that settles it." This is not a true saying. It should be, "God said it, and that settles it." When God speaks it is settled, whether we believe it or not. "He that believeth on the Son hath everlasting life: and he that believeth not the Son shall not see life; but the wrath of God abideth on him" (John 3:36). "Neither is there salvation in any other: for there is none other name under heaven given among men, whereby we must be saved" (Acts 4:12). "Jesus saith unto him, I am the way, the truth, and the life: no man cometh unto the Father, but by me" (John 14:6).

That settles it!

My prayer is that not one person will wake up in hell saying, "I did it my way." Salvation is not like an egg. I heard an egg can be used over one hundred different ways. It can be fried, boiled, poached, scrambled, and added raw to other ingredients to make cakes, cookies, cornbread, meatloaf, sauces, ice cream, etc. There are some who if God gave one hundred ways to salvation, they would want one hundred and one ways. Salvation is only by one way; it is God's love that is limitless. A children's song says, "One door and only one, but yet its sides are two. Inside and outside, on which side are you?" Salvation is by faith only in the finished work of Jesus Christ on Calvary for everyone.

Remember in your prayer life God answers prayers in different ways. First, God always answers someone who is repentant and wants to receive this great salvation instantly. After we become a born-again believer, he will answer our prayers in one of four different ways: (1) a direct answer, (2) a delayed answer, (3) a different answer, or (4) a denied answer. Whichever way he answers, we must accept his will. Our prayers may not be answered because we are not abiding in him. "If ye abide in me, and my words abide in you, ye shall ask what ye will, and it shall be done unto you" (John 15:7). That is a conditional verse. We need to abide in him, not get saved then continue to live for the things of this world, but abide, stay close, and obey. "And whatsoever we ask, we receive of him, because we keep his commandments, and do those things that are pleasing in his sight" (1 John 3:22). "And this is the confidence that we have in him, that, if we ask anything according to his will, he heareth us" (1 John 5:14). If we are abiding in him, we will not ask frivolously for unnecessary wants but for those things that will be pleasing to him, although there is nothing wrong with asking for some wants.

My valley at this time is breast cancer. Are you going through a valley at this moment? These principles hold true to anything that we may go through in life. Just depend on him, for he is the only one who knows the future! If we know of someone going through a crisis or difficult time, we need to stand by and support one another.

Alice Fletcher

Scientists have discovered some fascinating attributes of the geese. When geese fly in V formation, the goose in front, as he flaps his wings, causes an uplift for the one immediately behind, causing a greater flying range than if flying alone. If one goose leaves the formation, he will immediately feel a drag and quickly get back into formation. When the head goose gets tired, he will fall back and another goose will take the lead. The honking of the geese is to encourage the ones ahead to keep up the speed. If one leaves the formation, because of sickness or being wounded, two others will follow to give help and protection. You can see how they support, encourage, protect, and depend on each other. These are great lessons for us to learn.

On the lighter side, have you ever wondered why one side of the V formation is longer than the other? Someone recently pointed this out to me and gave a reason. There are more geese on one side than the other side! Seriously, I don't think science has figured that one out yet.

I must admit, while going through treatments, my mind did not dwell on cancer, but it seems I am more mindful of cancer returning now. I think it is based on the report that stated my cancer was aggressive. I pray for continual good health, and if cancer, or any other valley, occurs, I know it will be for a greater purpose. Some things in life we have no control over. Any valley I go through may be that God is preparing for me a deeper valley, so deep that church, preachers, family, or friends can't help—the only help will come straight from God. We must realize there are worse things in this world. Instead of magnifying our problems, we must magnify Jesus. Praise him for what we are going through, because through each valley we are being conformed to the image of his Son, if we submit to God's will. "And we know that all things work together for good to them that love God, to them who are the called according to his purpose. For whom he did foreknow, he also did predestinate to be conformed to the image of his Son ... " (Romans 8:28–29). I have found in my weakness, he is strong. I realize there are times when fear comes into our life, but when we experience that fear, we need to dwell on the following: "What time I am afraid, I will trust in thee" (Psalms 56:3). God's arm is not shortened where he cannot reach out and touch us.

As I was walking out of my valley back up to the mountaintop, where I would love to be at all times, he was by my side. When the Lord sees fit for me to go back through a valley, I know there will be greater lessons to learn. A past pastor, Dr. Charles E. Wright, a very devout man full of wisdom, said this many years ago, and it has stayed with me: "Lilies grow in the valley, not on the mountaintop." We mature and grow spiritually when we are in the valley. "He sendeth the springs into the valleys, which run among the hills," to refresh and cause us to flourish (Psalm 104:10). He is that living water that our soul thirsts for. So when you are in that valley in your life, you can still count it all joy, because if you treat your valley as a spiritual experience, you know you will be able to withstand the test and increase in the knowledge of the Lord.

Alice Fletcher

Where the Lilies Grow

Up upon the mountaintop is where I love to be,
Up where life is full of contentment
    and all is trouble-free.

When the inevitable tribulations come
    and I descend into
A valley, with him I have the power to stand.
Remembering 'tis God's promise
    to me that nothing
Nor anyone will be able to pluck me
    out of his hand.

On the day I find myself feeling in solitude down in
The lowest valley where the springs of water flow,
"I will lift up mine eyes unto the hills, from
    whence cometh my help,
My help cometh from the Lord," this assurance I know.

On top of the mountain I have joy unspeakable
As I find myself at my very best.
But when in the valley I can still count it all joy for
God said I will be able to withstand any test.

I will not remain on the mountaintop;
    on that pinnacle
I cannot forever reside.
As I travel down into the valley,
    I have the promise that
There with me he will also faithfully abide.

Out of my Valley

Preferring the mountaintop where the refreshing
    breezes blow,
I must ne'er forget, 'tis in the valley where the lilies grow.

John 10:28
Psalm 121:1

Can I Remain on the Mountaintop?

Everyone will go through trials, tribulation, and tough times in their life. There are many avenues that will take us through them. You may call them trials, storms, valleys, troubles, or whatever, but they are destined to come. No one will always have the perfect, peaceful life. "Many are the afflictions of the righteous: but the Lord delivereth him out of them all" (Palms 34:19). So, why do these appear out of nowhere?

God will never tempt us to do anything that is contrary to his word, but he will put us to a test to show our faithfulness to him or to bring us out of our slackness of fellowship to cause us to be closer to him. When these tribulations come, it is then we should realize it is for a purpose and we need to examine ourselves and see where we stand with him.

He will also chastise us for the sin in our life. It could be that he will single us out so he can show others what he can do through our lives, as they witness his workings in us.

Satan is the one that tempts us into sin against God. When we listen to the voice of Satan and follow after our own lust, that is when we find ourselves in the storms of life. Satan knows his destiny, and he wants everyone to reside in hell with him. After we are born again and are guaranteed our home in heaven, he wants us to live a defeated life and still follow his ways, although he knows we will never reside in hell with him. He knows he can no longer have our soul, but he wants to destroy our testimony and joy. The devil wants us to dwell in the past. Why should we stay in the past when God has removed all our sin from us, "As far as the east is from the west, so far hath he removed our transgressions from us" (Psalm 103:12). He not only removes them but also forgets them. "This is the covenant that I will make with them after those days, saith the Lord, I will put my laws into their hearts, and in their minds will I write them; And their sins and iniquities will I remember no more" (Hebrews 10:16–17).

The testing of God or the following of Satan's wooing both can lead us into these valleys.

Not all trials are a result from sin, but they are there for a purpose. We should not ask God, "Why me?" Ask, "Lord, what am I to learn from this?"

"My brethren, count it all joy when ye fall into divers temptations; Knowing this, that the trying of your faith worketh patience" (James 1:2–3).

Not all tribulations are primarily attributed to us personally. Think of the disasters that occur around the world and the devastation they bring, such as hurricanes, tornadoes, wild fires, tsunamis, earthquakes, etc. We may live in one of these areas where just by happenstance they occur, or God may send these to bring an awakening to a particular area. We may just happen to be in that area of judgment and have to face the results the disaster brings.

Many accounts in the Bible attest to this. God makes the way rough for someone to make his purpose to come about. Remember the life of Joseph in Genesis Chapter 37:39–50. Joseph was hated by his brothers, and, because of jealousy, they sold him to the Midianite merchantmen that were traveling through their land. The Midianites sold him in Egypt unto Potipher, an officer of Pharoah. Potipher noticed that in all Joseph did he was prosperous and the Lord was with him, so he made him overseer of his house. Potipher's wife, day after day, tried to seduce Joseph to no avail. One day she took him by his garment and he hastily departed, leaving her holding it. She was furious and lied to her husband, telling him Joseph tried to seduce her. Potipher believed his wife and had Joseph thrown into prison. He remained there falsely for two years, but the Lord was with Joseph and showed him mercy. Because of Joseph's testimony, Pharoah honored him by releasing him from prison and putting him into the position of being the second highest in Egypt, saying, "Only in the throne will I be greater than thou." Because of this tragedy that happened to Joseph, Israel was blessed. A famine came to the land, and all the kinsmen of Joseph came to Egypt to escape the famine. Through this, God's purpose for Israel's future was fulfilled, although they served as slaves four hundred and thirty years.

There may be someone close to us that is the reason for our troubles. Remember the account of Achan in Joshua 7. Israel lost the battle against Ai, and thirty-six men lost their lives. Joshua fell down before God and asked why. God told him because one in his army had disobeyed and had taken the spoils of the enemy at the battle of Jericho. "…There is an accursed thing in the midst of thee, O Israel: thou can't not stand before thine enemy until ye take away the accursed thing from among you" (Joshua 7:13). Achan took from the enemy those things that were pleasing to him, after God told the people to not bring anything back from the battle. He hid the goods under the floor of his tent. No one knew; only God alone knew. Not only was he under the punishment of God, but those of his household were also. After Achan's sin was made public and God's punishment came to him, God gave Israel the victory over Ai when they went into battle again against them. If we know of something going on in the confines of our home that is not acceptable to God, it should be addressed and immediately corrected before God has to do the correcting.

When the death door appears to someone we dearly love and we are going through this valley, we should not get mad with God for taking our loved one. God is the only one who holds the timetable of every life. In our sorrow of heart, we should remember that death appears anywhere in the span of life between life before birth up through someone past the century year. God alone is the decider of what time death will occur. "For my thoughts are not your thoughts, neither are your ways my ways, saith the Lord. For as the heavens are higher than the earth, so are my ways higher than your ways, and my thoughts than your thoughts" (Isaiah 55:8–9).

When a murder or fatal accident occurs, it may not be God's perfect will but his permissive will. I have seen many times when a tragedy like this happens to bring some of those acquainted to that person to realize life on earth is not forever. They realize their stand with God is not as it should be then accept Jesus as their Savior. We cannot always know nor understand the ways of God, only accept them. God can heal in times of sorrow. We must always be ready for the unexpected.

> In those days was Hezekiah sick unto death. And Isaiah the prophet the son of Amoz came unto him, and said unto him, Thus saith the Lord, Set thine house in order: for thou shalt die, and not live. Then Hezekiah turned his face toward the wall, and prayed unto the Lord, and said, Remember now, O Lord, I beseech thee, how I have walked before thee in truth and with a perfect heart, and have done that which is good in thy sight. And Hezekiah wept sore. Then came the word of the Lord to Isaiah, saying, Go, and say to Hezekiah, Thus saith the Lord, the God of David thy father, I have heard thy prayer, I have seen thy tears: behold I will add unto thy days fifteen years.
>
> Isaiah 38:1–5

No matter how upright in heart one is, it does not exempt them from sickness and death. God did restore his health as well as extend his days by fifteen years. If in your infirmities you pray as Hezekiah did but do not get the answer he did, just keep in mind God's grace is sufficient.

The season in the valley will not remain forever. When we find ourselves traveling back up to the mountaintop, we should give God praise and enjoy our stay up there for, in this world of woes, it may not be but a short time before we find ourselves headed back down into the valley. It is when we are in the valleys that we best examine ourselves, because when we are on the mountaintop we are in a state of contentment and satisfaction. We can prolong our stay on the mountain-top by daily Bible reading, prayer, memorizing Scripture, and a commitment to living our life that will be pleasing to our Lord, although these four basics will not keep anyone from going back down off the mountaintop. "But the land, whither ye go to possess it, is a land of hills and valleys, and drinketh water of the rain of heaven: A land which the Lord thy God careth for: the eyes of the Lord thy God are always upon it, from the beginning of the year even unto the end of the year" (Deuteronomy 11:11–12).

God is telling the Israelites about the Promised Land. The Promised Land to us is a picture of the consecrated life, one that is not lived in doing as the non-Christians of the world live. It cannot be a picture of heaven, as some believe, because there were still battles, death, heartaches, troubles, etc., which were present in the Promised Land that are not present in heaven. He is telling his people there will be val-leys as well as hills in their journeys, but he will always have his eyes upon them.

Think of the Apostle Paul in 2 Corinthians 12 and his

thorn in the flesh. He sought the Lord three times, that it might be removed. But God's answer was, "My grace is sufficient for thee." And Paul's reply was, "Most gladly therefore will I rather glory in my infirmities, that the power of Christ may rest upon me." The Bible does not tell us what his infirmity was for a reason. Further Scripture reveals his eyesight was very bad. Many believe this was his thorn in the flesh. There are those that develop an incurable disease that only God can heal or accidents that render one disabled. It is not God's will that everyone be healed, but his grace is sufficient for any situation. Having to live with an incurable disease or disability, God will give the mental ability, patience, and grace by measure that will sustain one through it.

Have you ever thought that maybe after we have been on the mountaintop for a season and begin to get high-minded God has to take us down so we will see him as he is, and he has to kick us off our high horse causing us to realize we need to depend on him and not on our own strength?

God always keeps his promises. It is ourselves that cause him to withhold from us because we do not keep the conditions that go along with the promises. Many promises in the Bible have a condition to go along with them. Example: "Draw nigh to God, and he will draw nigh to you ... " (James 4:8). When we come to realize that we are not as close to God as we have been in the past, guess which one of us has moved? God is always as near as we allow him to be.

God is so faithful. There is a scripture for every situation we may find ourselves in. The Syrian army had fought against Israel and lost. They were preparing to return for battle against them again.

And the servants of the king of Syria said unto him, Their gods are gods of the hills; therefore they were stronger than we; but let us fight against them in the plains, and surely we shall be stronger than they.

> 1 Kings 20:23

And there came a man of God, and spake unto the king of Israel, and said, Thus saith the Lord, Because the Syrians have said, The Lord is God of the hills, but he is not God of the valleys, therefore will I deliver all this great multitude into thine hand and ye shall know that I am the Lord.

> 1 Kings 20:28

Our enemy, Satan, tries to defeat us when we are in the valley, but " … we are more than conquerors through him that loved us (Romans 8: 37). Truly God is the God of the valleys as well as the mountains.

If we are not in a valley at this present time, it is inevitable we will be there at some point in time. When we find ourselves in the valley, remember: "I will lift up mine eyes unto the hills, from whence cometh my help. My help cometh from the Lord, which made heaven and earth" (Psalm 121:1–2).

When speaking of valleys, one can never forget Job.

There was a man … whose name was Job; and that man was perfect and upright, and one that feared God, and eschewed evil. And there were born unto him seven sons and three daughters. His substance also was seven thousand sheep, and three thousand camels, and five hundred yoke of oxen, and five hundred she asses, and a very great household: so that this man was the greatest of all the men of the east.

Job 1:1–3

And the Lord said unto Satan, Hast thou considered my servant Job, that there is none like him in the earth, a perfect and an upright man, one that feareth God, and escheweth evil? Then Satan answered the Lord, and said, Doth Job fear God for nought? Hast not thou made an hedge about him, and about his house, and about all that he hath on every side? Thou hast blessed the work of his hands, and his substance is increased in the land. But put forth thine hand now, and touch all that he hath, and he will curse thee to thy face. And the Lord said unto Satan. Behold, all that he hath is in thy power: only upon himself put not forth thine hand. So Satan went forth from the presence of the Lord.

Job 1:8–12

So, in one day Job lost all ten of his children, all of his livestock, and there came a great wind and smote the four corners of the house, and it fell. Did Job curse God? No.

Then Job arose, and rent his mantle, and shaved his head, and fell down upon the ground, and worshipped, and said, naked came I out of my mother's womb, and naked shall I return thither: the Lord gave, and the Lord hath taken away; blessed be the name of the Lord.

Job 1:20–21

And the Lord said unto Satan, Hast thou considered my servant Job, that there is none like him in the earth, a perfect and an upright man, one that feareth God and escheweth evil? And still he holdeth fast his integrity, although thou movedst me against him, to destroy him without cause. And Satan answered the Lord, and said, Skin for skin, yea, all that a man hath will he give for his life. But put forth thine hand now, and touch his bone and his flesh, and he will curse thee to thy face. And the Lord said unto Satan, Behold, he is in thine hand; but save his life. So went Satan forth from the presence of the Lord, and smote Job with sore boils from the sole of his foot unto his crown.

Job 2:3–7

Job's answer to his wife, who told him to curse God and die, was, "… What? shall we receive good at the hand of God, and shall we not receive evil? In all this did not Job sin with his lips" (Job 2:10). God's eyes were upon Job and saw his faithfulness and therefore blessed him and restored back to him double. "… also the Lord gave Job twice as much as he had before" (Job 42:10). Including giving him ten more children. "He had also seven sons and three daughters" (Job 42:13). God did not give him twice the number of children back because Job still had his ten children that died, although they were in the presence of God.

This was a test of Job's faith. Satan's goal was for Job to quit serving God. When we go through these trials, we should count it all joy because God has a plan for us. Anytime we fail, we deny the faith. How many of us have had such a day as Job? No, not one! "Man that is born of a woman is of few days, and full of trouble" (Job 14:1). God will only allow as much as we are able to handle by depending on him. Many cannot handle situations because they have not the peace and strength that can only be obtained through God. They depend on their own strength that is weak and vulnerable.

First Corinthians 10:13 is a verse everyone should memorize. I totally see why this was the first scripture Dan Harden gave me to memorize. "There hath no temptation taken you but such as is common to man: but God is faithful, who will not suffer you to be tempted above that ye are able; but will with the temptation also make a way to escape, that ye may be able to bear it" (1 Corinthians 10:13).

This verse tells us trials are universal and common to everyone, they are certain to come, God is with us, and they are escapable and limited to what we are able to sustain.

To answer the question of the chapter title, no, we cannot remain on the mountaintop forever. I expect to traverse back down the mountain side again, but in the small Old Testament book of the prophets, it says, "The Lord is good, a strong hold in the day of trouble; and he knoweth them that trust in him" (Nahum 1:7). Everyone will go through tough times. God uses the tough times to bring beauty to the soul that nothing else can. It is just phenomenal how the Lord works in our lives. It is only God that can make the crooked way straight and the rough way smooth!

Whether on the mountaintop or plunged into the deepest valley, God has told us, "Speaking to yourselves in psalms and hymns and spiritual songs, singing and making melody in your heart to the Lord; Giving thanks always for all things unto God and the Father in the name of our Lord Jesus Christ" (Ephesians 5:19–20). Giving thanks for all things, not just for the wonderful things, sounds impossible when you are in the trials and valleys of life. But God said this; therefore, it is attainable. "I will bless the Lord at all times: his praise shall continually be in my mouth" (Psalms 34:1). "Let every thing that hath breath praise the Lord. Praise ye the Lord" (Psalm 150:6). "The dead praise not the Lord ..." (Psalm 115:17). Therefore, the conclusion is if you are not dead but living and have breath, you should be praising the Lord at all times.

+ In your happy moments ... thank God.
+ In your difficult moments ... seek God.
+ In your quiet moments ... worship God.
+ In your painful moments ... trust God.
+ In your every moment ... praise God.

Since we can be in the presence of God at all times, why not praise him continually? We need to have joy in our hearts that only comes from him. There is a difference between joy and happiness. Happiness comes from our circumstances and can be extinguished when difficult things happen. But joy can remain even in those troubled times, because we know God is our Father and he has permitted the troubles and will be with us through them. True joy only comes from hearing, reading, believing, and obeying the Word of God. I know there are some who are in a valley that is a permanent situation, as one having a permanent disability or illness, or one taking care of such a one that has been that way since birth or after an accident. This to me would be extremely devastating, but God has promised he would not give us more than we can handle, and still in all things we are to give thanks and praise.

Sometimes we can't handle the task at hand on our own but must reach out to others to help us along the way. It is not a shameful thing to admit you need help from others, although I have the personality that I don't like others to help and want to do everything on my own. God is able to change that and give us the desire for others to help. "I have shewed you all things, how that so labouring ye ought to support the weak, and to remember the words of the Lord Jesus, how he said, It is more blessed to give than to receive" (Acts 20:35). If we refuse help from someone or refrain from asking for the support, we cause someone else to not receive a blessing from the Lord as they minister to us.

As I was writing this, the Lord brought to mind something that happened thirty-three years ago for an example. Young mothers of today, there was a time when we used cloth diapers that had to be washed, dried on the clothesline, and folded. Our fourth son was only a few weeks old, and a lady from the church came by to visit. I had taken the diapers off the line and brought them inside just prior to her arrival, and they were on the couch unfolded. She so graciously offered to fold them but I refused. I know the Lord blessed her for the offer, but I did not receive the blessing by allowing her do it. Oh, how we cause sadness to the Lord in such little ways. If we joyfully accept help from others, we are both blessed.

As you can see, we cause the Lord to withhold his blessings from us at times. In one of my difficult times, as I was recovering from childbirth and maintaining a household, the Lord sent help, which I did not receive. By receiving the help, we both could have been praising the Lord, but I put a damper on things.

Praising the Lord in troubled times is something that needs to be trained for. We need to draw a line on some things and train for the desires of God. To learn to praise the Lord in bad times may have to start with a stumped toe. No matter how bad it hurts, we give praise to him that we did not hurt the whole foot. If you are traveling in your vehicle and run over something in the road and have a flat tire, praise the Lord for it, as it may have kept you from being in a severe accident further down the road.

I remember a time we were traveling through Florida, and just before an exit ramp off the interstate, the temperature gauge in our car showed the car was running hot. Ed pulled off at the ramp into a service station immediately and had the problem fixed in a short time. As we proceeded back onto the interstate, there was a sign that showed the next exit was forty-eight miles away. Tell me that was not a time to praise the Lord.

As you master praising the Lord for things such as this, you advance to praising him for greater things. Praising the Lord in all things has to start out with the little things, just as a baby must learn to take baby steps before he can learn to run. Surely you don't think in Job's situation that was the first time he had praised the Lord.

Out of my Valley

Although the fig tree shall not blossom, neither shall fruit be in the vines; the labour of the olive shall fail, and the fields shall yield no meat; the flock shall be cut off from the fold, and there shall be no herd in the stall: Yet I will rejoice in the Lord, I will joy in the God of my salvation.

Habakkuk 3:17–18

You can't have this cheer in your life until you know the one that brings cheer. I know there may be someone thinking, *But you don't know my situation! I am at a point where I don't have anywhere else to go.* There is always God. You may be so overwhelmed and confused you feel like you are at the end, but God says when you can't do anything else, just stand. "Wherefore take unto you the whole armour of God, that ye may be able to withstand in the evil day, and having done all, to stand. Stand therefore ... " (Ephesians 6:13–14). You feel as though you have done all you can do; what now? Just stand, do nothing else, and tell God you have done all; everything else is left up to him. Most of the time we try to work things out on our own.

This saith the Lord, Let not the wise man glory in his wisdom, neither let the mighty man glory in his might, let not the rich man glory in his riches: But let him that glorieth glory in this, that he understandeth and knoweth me, that I am the Lord which exercise lovingkindness, judgment, and righteousness in the earth: for in these things I delight, saith the Lord.

Jeremiah 9:23–24

We need to listen to God, for he is serious in his relationship with us! His way of communicating with us is through his Word, first by receiving salvation, by correction, and by his promises. Sometimes we have to change our behavior to accept the promise. Some conditional promises in his Word are, "My son, forget not my law; but let thine heart keep my commandments: For length of days, and long life, and peace, shall they add to thee" (Proverbs 3:1–2). "He that dwelleth in the secret place of the most High shall abide under the shadow of the Almighty" (Psalm 91:1). Also, "The Lord is on my side: I will not fear: what can man do unto me?" (Psalm 118:6). Our only hope is in our Lord, "Which hope we have as an anchor of the soul, both sure and stedfast..." (Hebrews 6:19). "Who shall separate us from the love of Christ? shall tribulation, or distress, or persecution, or famine, or nakedness, or peril, or sword?... Nay, in all these things we are more than conquerors through him that loved us" (Romans 8:35–37).

Since this is the day the Lord hath made, we need to listen to what he has for us today from his Word and refuse to let our circumstances get bigger than our God. When we have pain in our body, we know something is wrong and we can seek help; it's the same thing with pain in our soul, and we need help that only comes from him. With all that our Savior is, how can we not praise him for everything! The holy, almighty God alone is worthy of all praise. Those two words we don't hear much of today—holy and almighty. If we keep in mind the magnificence of it all, we will stay in a constant state of praise.

We need to concentrate on, "all things work together for

good." I told Marianne she had my permission to thank the Lord for my cancer, for if it was not for mine she would not have sought out my doctor when she did to discover her cancer. If she prolonged having her mammogram, it would have been in a more serious stage by the time she did so.

Did you know the trees and mountains and hills have the ability to praise our God? "For ye shall go out with joy, and be led forth with peace: the mountains and the hills shall break forth before you into singing, and all the trees of the field shall clap their hands" (Isaiah 55:12). Therefore, having this eternal life through the shed blood of Jesus Christ, how much the more should we be praising him? "By him therefore let us offer the sacrifice of praise to God continually, that is, the fruit of our lips giving thanks to his name" (Hebrews 13:15). "I will sing unto the Lord as long as I live: I will sing praise to my God while I have my being" (Psalm 104:33). When Jesus was making his triumphant entry into Jerusalem where he was to be crucified and the multitude were praising him with loud voices, "some of the Pharisees from among the multitude said unto him, Master, rebuke thy disciples. And he answered and said unto them, I tell you that, if these should hold their peace, the stones would immediately cry out" (Luke 19:39–40). I don't want the stones to replace me and my responsibility.

Our past pastor's wife, Trish McCoy, said the following statement that is so profound and should make one stop and think. "If God took everything away from you that you have not praised and thanked him for, how much would you lose?"

The second verse Dan Harden gave me to memorize back

in July 1970 is, "But sanctify the Lord God in your hearts: and be ready always to give an answer to every man that asketh you a reason of the hope that is in you with meekness and fear" (1 Peter 3:15).

Through this memoir, I pray I have shown you the reason of the hope that is in me and displayed the goodness, kindness, healing hand, grace, and mercy of our omnipotent, omnipresent, and omniscient Lord. I hope that I have shown you that if you do not have the peace of salvation and presence from him you can receive it today.

In retrospect, talking about our eternal life through Jesus Christ and praising him for all things, I want to share a little story I heard. Even more reason to praise him for things to come.

There was a woman who had a terminal illness and was given only a few months to live. She called her pastor to make final arrangements. She planned her own funeral, what songs she wanted sung, what scripture she wanted read, and what dress she wanted to be buried in. She also requested to be buried with her Bible in her left hand. One more thing, she wanted a fork to be in her right hand. As she saw the shocked look on her pastor's face, she went on to say how she had enjoyed the church fellowships and banquets and as the dinner plates were being cleared away someone would always say for those in attendance to keep their fork. She knew the best was on the way; the delicious desserts were the next thing on the menu. Her pastor made sure her wishes were carried through when the time came. At the viewing he watched as the room was abuzz with everyone talking about the fork in her hand, and he could not wait for the funeral service to explain. At her service, with all her wishes having been fulfilled, he began to explain the reason for the fork. With tears welled up in his eyes, he told of the lady's great faith and her assurance that heaven would be her eternal home. The fork represented better things to come. The fork and its meaning had a great impact on everyone. Now, as you are holding your fork, remember this: The best is yet to come!

Alice Fletcher

Don't Let the Stones Cry Out

T'was a time in my life when I was unfulfilled and lost;
I searched among the pleasures of this world at any cost.
Finding nothing in this world that could
    satisfy my soul,
Then I found Jesus who filled that emptiness
    and made me whole.

Because he transformed me from death unto life,
Brought me forth out of my world of strife,
As I continually worship him with my
    praise and adoration,
I will forever be thankful for his love and
    this so great salvation.

When I am in the deepest valley and I don't
    know what to do,
I'll praise him believing he can restore and
    make all things new.
Or sailing along peacefully then finding
    myself on the stormy sea,
Keeping in mind 'tis in the storm he
    is in the midst of it with me.

I am forever safe in the shadow of his
    almighty hand,
Whether up on the mountain or deep valley
    in this weary land.
I am compelled to praise my Creator, Savior,
    and Provider above,
And never cease to forget his everlasting,
    abiding love.

Out of my Valley

I must praise him when things are peaceful
    for I surely know,
It won't be long before a crisis comes in
    this old world of woe.
In all things give thanks and praise,
    trusting him without a doubt,
Because Jesus said,
      "If these should hold their peace, the stones
      would immediately cry out."

Isaiah 51:16
Luke 19:40

O magnify the Lord with me, and let us exalt his name together.

Psalm 34:3

Only fear the Lord, and serve him in truth with all your heart: for consider how great things he hath done for you.

1 Samuel 12:24

The grace of the Lord Jesus Christ, and the love of God, and the communion of the Holy Ghost, be with you all. Amen.

2 Corinthians 13:14

He which testifieth these things saith, Surely I come quickly. Amen. Even so, come, Lord Jesus. The grace of our Lord Jesus Christ be with you all. Amen.

Revelation 22:20–21

Out of my Valley

The Bible Memory Association mentioned in the first chapter is no longer known by that name. It is known as:

Scripture Memory Fellowship, Int.

P.O. Box 411551

St. Louis, MO 63141

www.scripturememoryfellowship.org